# Qigong for Beginners

## YOUR PATH TO GREATER HEALTH & VITALITY

DAVID J. COON

# CONTENTS

# DEDICATION

First, I dedicate this book to all my teachers who were kind enough to share their secret knowledge of the ages with me. Second, I dedicate this book to the teachers and students who have asked me to share that knowledge far and wide.

# ACKNOWLEDGMENTS

I want to thank my teachers who have carried on and passed on the torch to me so that all beings may become free. I want to thank my biological mom for her unstoppable character and her rebellious nature. I thank her for her love and for being an impetus to my martial arts training that led me to qigong. I want to thank my father for his love and his ability to communicate with and serve the public and for the art of running. I want to thank my grandfather, who is now on the other side, for his love, intensity, strength, and fortitude. I want to thank him for teaching me to walk around obstacles or—when that wasn't possible—to go through them. I want to thank my grandmother for her great love and support. I want to thank my brother for our ongoing, growing, and evolving friendship and I am so happy he has discovered Grace. Thank you Grace, so happy to have you in our family.

I want to thank my extended family, especially Gail, Len, Leslie, and Kristen Farnsworth, aka the Farnsworths. It was short, but I have great memories and I appreciate you all. I want to thank Ken Grider for all the time we've spent downloading the truth and sharing many moments of great laughter.

I want to thank my friend John Oliver for his friendship, his *soul* support, his presence, and his profound connection to the light! I want to thank Jerhoam—my gratitude is beyond words. I want to thank my sangha friends who I feel like I have known for eons. I want to thank Linda for her support of the great work and her great efforts to embody the teachings I have been involved in over the years.

I want to thank all of my students and clients from around the country and beyond. You placed your faith in me and the knowledge I carry and dared to apply the teachings, the techniques, the philosophies, the ancient sciences, and the theories to your lives. Without you and your willingness I could not possibly be where I am today.

I want to thank Tanya, my beloved wife, and Bella, my beloved daughter, who have worked beside me and dedicated themselves to getting this vital information into the hands, hearts, and minds of many people. I want to thank Tanya for her incredible dedication and effort in rain, cold, and shine. I want to thank her for all of the foundational details, organization, planning, and fundraising that goes into making these teachings accessible as continuing education for professionals like acupuncturists and massage therapists, as well as for the general public. Tanya's creativity and genius as an acupuncturist, president of Qigong Awareness, graphic designer, marketer, etc., etc., etc., have contributed greatly (times ten!) to the work.

I also want to thank Tanya for her creative genius, love, and support. I want to thank my daughter Bella for being an amazing light being whose presence graces Tanya and me in both work and in play. I want to thank Bella for sharing her daddy with the world on the weekends and many hours of the day during the week. I appreciate her willingness to work alongside her mom and me as we continue to metaphorically and quite literally take her homeschooling on the road.

I want to thank Sharon Chung for her faith in, belief in, and support of this great work, which she has demonstrated in a multitude of ways over the years. She has been instrumental in moving Qigong Awareness forward and getting these teachings out into the world. I also want to thank her for supporting my family and her family. She has given all the children someone to look up to and emulate, and I thank her especially for her love and service to all of them.

I want to thank our graphic designer Kristen who has contributed greatly to the creation of our website, our marketing materials and now the cover and design of this book. Your work is amazing. I want to thank Murphy at Kudzu Branding for the photos and for the inspirational powwows about branding and marketing. I want to give a big thanks to my editor, who I feel like I have known for a long, long time, Maureen McIntyre. I want to thank her for joining me in the great work and putting these teachings out into the world for the benefit of all sentient beings. I believe her great skills as the chief editor of this book and her help in communicating these teachings to the reader in a clear and concise fashion will help many people, many souls. Your talents are greatly appreciated! Many thanks for joining me in this endeavor.

I want to thank Kaitlyn Moore for her proofreading and her editing skills. Your work, suggestions, and efforts are so much appreciated. Many thanks!

I want to thank Mark Pergola for his dedication and follow-through with some of our initial qigong videos and online courses. Great work! Thanks to modern technology, we are reaching people around the world.

Thank you to my uncles Len Banach and Tom Brett who helped me to see that having your own business was better than working for somebody else. Uncle Len taught me about determination and using exercise as an outlet and driving force. Uncle Tom taught me to start my first business and he helped teach me that I never wanted to work for anyone else but myself and that I could one day become an entrepreneur. Thank you to the Brett clan as well, much love to all.

I also want to specifically thank Harvey and Anna Chung for their support of our work over the years. Much thanks to the Scott and Lescault families for your love and support.

To my martial arts students Jim, Dave, Bryan, Phoenix, Gabe, Tommy, Chris, Richie, Matt, and the many others I have trained in the early years, thank you. To Paul Z., my first martial arts master instructor, thank you. To Master Kwon, my Tae Kwon Do master, a huge thanks to you for your guidance in what it means to be a master and your great lessons about how to live life. To Ikeda sensei, my Aikido master, many thanks for your teachings about connection and *relax*ing the mind and body and your many words of wisdom. To Dr. Hou, one of my qigong master teachers, many thanks for your insights into the practice, and to Master Tam, many thanks to you as well for helping me kick-start my own path.

To my many students of *enlightenment* who have been willing to unearth themselves to find the light that lives within them, I am honored to be your soul guide and friend: Linda, Christa, Phil, Ting Ting, Yvette, Dr. Bill, Paul Solari, John Marquard, Gary B., Dr. Angie, Sandy, Maureen, Molly, Suzanne, Barbara,Sue, Mary, Brenda, Phyllis, Tracy, Sarah, Margo,

Simm, Jan, and Charlie and many, many others who have attended our workshops over the years.

Thanks to all the students who have come out to the live workshops and to our now Certified Qigong Instructors and Medical Qigong Practitioners. At the time of this writing, we have two fully Certified Qigong Instructors who are also fully Certified Medical Qigong Practitioners. (Linda and Yvette). We have more than twenty others following suit, and many more to come. Thank you to all of you who are contributing to our qigong network and Qigong Awareness family.

Many thanks to some of my teachers from the early years: Dr. Tolk, Dr. Austin, Dr. Bruce, and Master Silva, thank you to all. I want to thank Roianne for her healing skills and helping me to evolve myself and my work. I want to thank Chuck B. I want to thank my family friends the Servants. I want to thank Marky Younis and family for your friendship.

Lisa Siciliano thank you for the rock star photos that cover our website and facebook and some of which have made it into our ebook! You rock!

The list goes on, and I am sure I temporarily forgot some important names and people. I will be adding more over the years I am sure.

# AUTHOR'S BIO

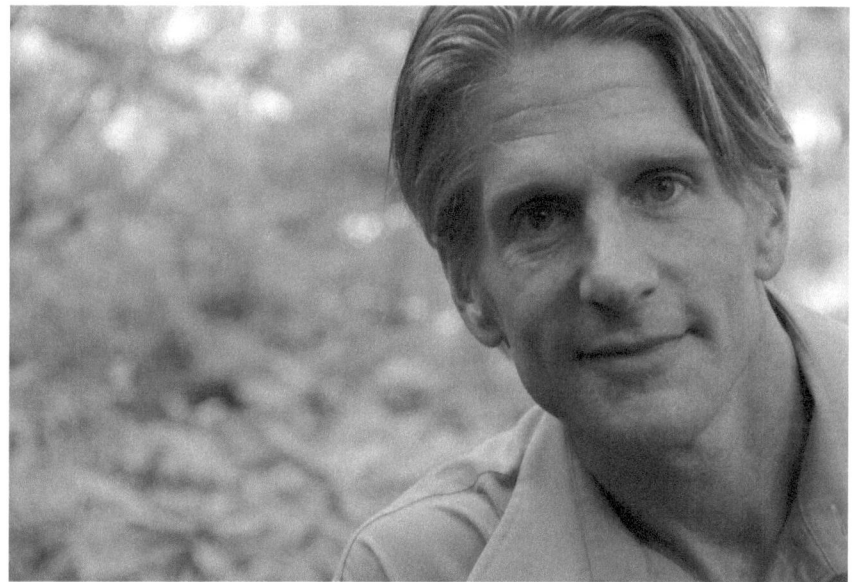

*Photo by: Murphy Funkhouser- Capps*

David J. Coon has been practicing qigong and medical qigong for over thirty years. David discovered qigong as a young teenager, and it allowed him to heal mental, emotional, and physical pain, as well as a severe spinal disease. David now teaches qigong and medical qigong around the country to lay people and professionals, sharing with them the healing power of the mind over matter. David is both an author and inspirational speaker. He currently resides with his wife and daughter in North Carolina.

# FOREWORD

I have known David Coon for more than 15 years and am excited that he has now written this book to complement his videos and other programs, both live and online.

I have personally and professionally benefited from his teachings and approach to medical qigong since I first attended his programs in Denver, Colorado, in 2003. David's approach is always inspirational because he brings such a level of energy, devotion, and commitment to the well-being of his students!

With David's help, I and many other students have learned qigong techniques in an enjoyable and effective manner. And this is so important, because qigong has so much to offer in providing benefits for improved health, reduced stress, and improved overall well-being!

I remember attending a program with David and fellow students in Boulder a number of years ago. David was leading the group breathing exercise and after a number of minutes I felt this surging rush of energy throughout my arms and body that I can only explain as a raging river of energy that was truly amazing! It was, needless to say, very profound, exhilarating, and unforgettable!

In my more than 45 years in medicine and healthcare, after graduating from the medical school at the Columbia University College of Physicians and Surgeons, I have always emphasized cellular health as the fundamental factor in promoting well-being and preventing disease. This means that the more we can provide oxygen and nutrients to the cells and the more we can activate the pathways for cellular detoxification, the healthier the body's 100 trillion cells will be. And healthier cells mean a healthier body!

This is what qigong exercises, done on a consistent basis, can provide—improved cellular health and greater flow of the life energy that organizes and orchestrates the countless biological functions that determine our health and well-being.

And then there are the mental, emotional and spiritual benefits of qigong, which impact our physical health through the mind-body connection. This is another area where Master David Coon excels! He teaches and demonstrates qigong from the heart and therefore creates a connection with his students that is truly profound.

I am looking forward to the expansion of David's work and know that those who participate in any of his programs will be deeply rewarded with many blessings.

Bill Bergman, M.D.
Naples, Florida
September 2017

# TESTIMONIALS

*David is a magic man!*

---

LISA SICILIANO,
Rock & Roll Photographer to the Stars

*I knew from reading David's Bio that he has extensive training in Qigong as well as other related experience. Personally I have trained with quite a few Qigong teachers over 13 years but nothing prepared me for what I experienced in person in his Medical Qigong training class.*

*The power of his energy is obvious and palpable. We were practicing poses which we held for an extended period and I was having spasms and cramping in my back and was breathing to release as instructed. I thought that I had reached my limit as the muscles began to lockup. David looked at me across the room and I could tell he recognized my situation and in an instant my spasm released and I could tell from his glance that he transmitted the energy which broke the cramping. This is a great course and he is not only an enthusiastic and talented instructor but obviously a powerful healer as well. Not to be missed. I cannot wait to complete the full Certification and am excited to see what is in the future.*

---

Leon Mckay LAc MATOM,
Qigong Instructor - Wilmington, NC

I have been training with David for almost a year now. When David moved to Wilmington, I had been practicing Qigong sporadically for a month or so with an instructor who was in David's certification program. Qigong seemed cool, but I had not had any previous experience with energy work and was, admittedly, skeptical. However, I had had breast cancer 3 times and was fed up with the options that Western medicine offered. I was overwhelmed with side effects and took a handful of pills a couple of times a day. When the cancer returned the third time, I was medical retired from the Army and my physical condition has deteriorated from being very physically fit to barely being able to walk a mile.

In the past year, I have trained with David in Qigong classes, Intensives, and private sessions, as well as participating in his healing clinics. Since beginning training, I have been able to stop taking 7 different prescription medications, lost 20 lbs., can run 5 miles, and am a certified Level 1 Qigong Instructor. The difference in my physical, emotional, and spiritual well being has been phenomenal. David is an amazing healer, instructor, and coach. My story for the past 8 years has been a story of cancer. **Thanks to David, my story is now a story of healing, health, and prosperity.**

MELISSA L. CULBRETH,
MDIV, MA, QI-50 - MAJOR-RETIRED, US ARMY,
QIGONG INSTRUCTOR Carolina Beach, NC

I recently participated in a weekend Medical Qigong Intensive with David Coon, and I returned to my practice full of life force and eager to assimilate my experience into my treatment approach. The sessions were well-organized and well-balanced between information and hands-on activities, reminding us that true qigong is something quite beyond exercise! I look forward to future workshops. David is a testament to his own mastery, and his commitment to practicing and teaching medical qigong may very well result in a resurrection in the United States of a much-neglected branch of Chinese medicine. We here in North Carolina are fortunate to have David and Tanya living in our area.

ROBIN R. WHITLOW,
Diplomate in Acupuncture, Diplomate in Chinese Herbology,
Licensed Acupuncturist, Hillsborough, North Carolina

*I met David Coon many years ago when he was teaching an introductory class on energy and healing. I took an instant liking to him and his unusual level of personal energy and integrity. Since then, I have had the honor of watching David, who was already a skilled practitioner, fine-tune and enhance his skills to a rather remarkable degree.*

***Among his many outstanding characteristics are his fierce dedication and determination to not only being the best that he himself can be, but to passing along the benefits of that intentional ethic to those fortunate enough to be taught or treated by him personally.*** *For David, being good has never been good enough. And, in my experience, it is quite unusual for a "healer"—of any kind—to not only always set the highest standards for their work, but to insist that they personally, continuously reach for an ever-higher level of attainment.*

*David has always studied healing, consciousness, and the nature of reality with outstanding diligence. Thus, he has come to know a great many things about the physical and energetic worlds, both within this universe and within each of us.* ***So, if you are seeking someone who is highly trained and will always give you the very best they have to offer, then David is one of the very best souls you could ever work with.***

PAUL SOLARI, M.A.,
Licensed Professional Counselor, Boulder, Colorado

***David Coon was instrumental in helping me win my first major golf tournament.*** *Originally, I had gone to David to help me with my physical pain, which he did. However, the techniques he taught me were not only helpful for that, but also allowed me to increase my focus and mental capabilities to perform at much higher levels as an athlete...I continue to use these techniques many years later to improve myself in all aspects of my life.*

GARY Borgese,
Boulder, Colorado

*I had an acute kidney infection with a high fever and, after checking with my doctor, I went to see David. He helped me to see all the false beliefs that I was holding on to. [During the session]...**I let go of all the stories I had been*** *telling myself with a great amount of laughter,* I woke up the next day symptom-free. Sent with love and gratitude!

---

LINDA WHILDIN,
Certified Massage Therapist, Boulder, Colorado

*It seems to me that one of the truly great ironies of life is that most of us spend our days stumbling about in a dream-like state, seeking happiness and fulfillment in the external world, and never realizing that deep inner peace is not only readily within our grasp, but is actually the essence of who we truly are. Coming to this realization is the first step in waking up, but the question becomes, "What is preventing us from accessing our natural state?" Admittedly, the process of self-realization must be a personal experience, but that does not mean that we cannot receive assistance and guidance from others.*

*I can say that qigong and the teachings transmitted through David Coon have truly helped me in the process of awakening, gaining better health, and experiencing deeper and more profound moments of peace. I had been doing qigong of sorts before I met David, but the practice took on dramatically new dimensions after I began studying with him.*

---

Phillip Chilson, Ph.D. (Physics),
Professor of Meteorology

*David's Medical Qigong Intensive workshop was superb!*

*He was extremely skilled at communicating concepts and ideas with insight and clarity. The activities he chose were very helpful and allowed each person to grow from their current place of understanding and level of skill. I personally came away from the workshop with a much greater depth of understanding that will inform my personal and professional practice. A couple of "nuggets" have already resulted from applying some of his suggestions. I heartily recommend this.*

---

DIANE GROSS,
Doctor of Oriental Medicine, Licensed Acupuncturist, author
of *The Art of Personal Alchemy: Transform Your Emotional
Lead into Gold*, Greensboro, North Carolina

*Who would studying with David be good for? Everyone!*

*As an acupuncturist, I found it ideal. That said, you do not need to have ANY concept of chi to take this course; if you simply believe your body has power, and your body has the capability to heal itself, then you're ready to start. For beginners, this course will start you on the path of mastering your bodily functions by introducing you to chi and providing you the daily tools and practices necessary to develop this ability. From there, it's up to you. For the seasoned practitioner, there is still great knowledge to glean from this course. David's discussions on the endocrine system and glands, their importance and relation to the chakras, the kundalini, the overall tie to the Caduceus symbol—I could go on, but he probably wouldn't appreciate me divulging the entire course. Let's put it this way—if I equate this course to the trunk of a tree, now that the course is completed, I have at least five different branches or pathways to explore further that I did not have before. I greatly appreciate the tidbits of information David left along the way that opened this door. My cup is full and I will spend the next several weeks, months, years, and decades digesting its contents.*

TIFFANY GAROFALO,
Licensed Acupuncturist, Layton, Utah

**As an acupuncturist, keeping up with continuing education unit requirements is sometimes a chore.** *On more than one occasion, I've sat through droning presentations of rehashed information, just hoping for something useful and watching the clock.* **Not so with David's qigong workshop! From the first moment to the last I was engaged and fascinated**, *with a hundred ideas running through my head about how to better help my patients. I know I have to cultivate my own practice first, but I've known that for a long time. After this seminar, I finally feel like I have a starting place and a foundation that will help me prioritize my own practice and slowly evolve into a better practitioner for my patients. Thanks David!*

ANAYA PALAY, DAOM,
Doctor of Acupuncture and
Oriental Medicine, Panama City

*David Coon is a true teacher.*

*His thorough discussions were filled with valuable information. His explanations throughout the class were both relatable and one step ahead of any question that may have arisen as he was teaching. I have since started my own qigong practice, and have incorporated medical qigong into my acupuncture practice.*

JODI ROSE, M.S.,
Licensed Acupuncturist, Brooklyn Heights NYC

*In coming to this Medical Qigong Intensive, **I was seeking a teacher with a genuine desire to share and guide in their knowledge and experiences, a teacher that exhibits true passion and a dedication to the art of qigong. Furthermore, someone who has a calm way of conveying, engaging and assisting all who are there in learning to cultivate chi for themselves as well as to help others.** It was a true pleasure to attend the Intensive and meet and learn from David, a qigong master who embodies all of the above. I look forward to the next qigong learning experience! With gratitude, Jeanie.*

JEANIE THAM,
Diplomate of Acupuncture and Oriental Medicine, Licensed Acupuncturist, Board-Certified Herbalist, New Jersey/New York

*The Golden Dragon Medical Qigong Intensive exceeded my expectations. **David is clearly a master.** The instructions and information given were grounded, thorough, and easy to understand and follow. **I came away feeling really inspired** to continue my practice and am reaping the benefits every day! Thanks for such a valuable, practice-enhancing and heart-centered course!*

SALLY ADAMS,
R.N. San Diego, California

*I have been in practice in the alternative health field as a doctor of chiropractic focusing on applied kinesiology, acupuncture and neuro-emotional technique for*

*34 years. I've also been a qigong student for 8 years. I highly recommend David Coon's workshops for anyone who is looking to deepen their understanding of qigong, further their own personal inward journey and provide benefit to others through the techniques that he teaches so masterfully. David is genuine and authentic, skilled and compassionate. It is a privilege to study with him.*

---

DR. T. HAMBRICK,
Chiropractic and Applied Kinesiology,
Clearwater, Florida

*David's Golden Dragon Medical Qigong Intensive was by far the most powerful and life-changing course I have taken.*

*My practice is already completely different in just the first day. And, my city must have gotten the memo because my clinic is 25% fuller this week than ever before.*

---

RHIANNON HUTTON,
Doctor of Chiropractic, Master of Acupuncture and Oriental Medicine, Licensed Acupuncturist, Fayetteville, North Carolina

*Being in David Coon's medical qigong class was an enlivening and fortifying experience for me. The practices taught were simple yet powerful. I returned to my life to find my way to the inner energy core of the exercises he shared with us. I particularly loved the integrity with which David teaches. He physically manifests a high mastery of martial arts and qigong. He did not try to make us learn what he did but encouraged us to find our own way to our own practice.*
***David is one of those rare teachers who has the charisma and capacity to empower his students** to encounter and channel their own power. **I walked away with a renewed commitment to qigong as a powerful medicine.** I renewed a connection in my own mind to practice regularly. Before, I practiced, but sporadically. David's passion made it clear to me that practice every day is as important as brushing my teeth or eating every day. A veil lifted and a strong sense of commitment rooted. It started with experiencing the power of standing posture. I understood power is revealed as you practice every day.*

*The classes that I have taken with David Coon are phenomenal!*

*They are easy to understand, fun, and have takeaway benefits that affect my life directly as well as all my clients in my massage practice. I will continue to take his classes whenever possible. I strongly suggest taking any class with this qigong master!*

KAY WISE-DENTY,
Licensed Massage and Bodywork Therapist,
Black Mountain, North Carolina

*David's healing seminar was like the Magical Mystery Tour of the breath and power of intent. David Coon has walked the walk and is **truly changing the planet with this message of breathing** and the ability to heal using qigong techniques.*

JEANNETTE FLOM,
Montessori directress and fitness
instructor, Tampa, Florida

*I participated in the The Golden Dragon Medical Qigong Intensive with David this last weekend in Clearwater/St. Petersburg. It was a very transformative experience for me. David is a "True Master of Qigong" who has the desire to fully engage his students, taking a very personal interest in the development of each and every one. He is a gifted instructor with a thorough understanding of qigong and the martial arts from many paths.*

*This weekend was very different. I have attended other qigong seminars in the past. They left me disenchanted, overwhelmed, and totally frustrated. I left these weekends without retaining anything from the class except a paper certificate stating that I had fulfilled my continuing education unit requirements for yet another year.*

***David's class brought me to a new level, demonstrating that I have the power to transform myself and become a healing channel through this practice.***

*I realize that to appreciate the power and art of qigong, I must practice daily. David communicated the qigong exercises and concepts in a way I could* understand so I could integrate the practice into my life and work. The way he led the class through the various exercises was clear and concise. The sessions were timed, organized, and well-balanced between informative experiential lectures and "hands-on" practical experience, reminding me that true qigong is more than a technique or modality, it is a gift! David repeatedly encouraged participants to "feel" the chi, not just apply yet another technique.

He truly left me inspired, with a desire to pursue a qigong path. This has been one of the best programs I have attended as a continuing education seminar. The class should be mandatory for every student of acupuncture and life. It is a fulfilling experience; I honestly recommend his medical intensive for everyone to attend. I look forward to future workshops and continued practice.

WES EADES,
Acupuncture Physician (Florida), Diplomate in Acupuncture,
National Certification Board for Therapeutic Massage and
Bodywork, Acupuncture Wellness LLC, Lady Lake, Florida

I walked away from this workshop feeling so empowered. I went home feeling grounded, strong, and enlightened. I am a licensed acupuncturist, and the workshop has totally changed my practice. I am more present during treatments and my intuition has expanded. **I am looking forward to the next class because this one has totally changed my life.**

MARCY L'HOMMEDIEU,
Licensed Acupuncturist and Massage Therapist, Savannah, Georgia

I've been around energy medicine for 35 years. As a practitioner of Chinese medicine, I've had the opportunity to study with many teachers. David Coon takes the lead in having mastered qigong practices. His mastery extends to his ability to share his techniques and practices in exercises and routines that are simple to implement and use. I have done from five minutes to as much as a one-hour practice in the morning.

Sometimes I integrate the practices into my day. The results have amazed me. My physical endurance, inner calm, clarity, and intuition are optimal. **I highly** *recommend Qigong Awareness to anyone of any age looking for a better quality of life. I am grateful for the privilege of having David Coon as a teacher.*

JACOB BARROCAS,
Mentor, Coach, Consultant, Author

*After an ultrasound and MRI (July 9–10, 2017), I was strongly advised to have my gall bladder removed by my primary physician and GI specialist. Luckily, the surgeon re-reviewed the MRI and informed my primary physician that the surgery was not urgent. In parallel that week, I fasted, meditated, and practiced Qigong. **David's weekend seminar was striking in that I felt a palpable acceleration in my healing and a return to strength.***

*My blood retest a few weeks later showed a dramatic return to normal liver functions. **My primary physician was nothing less than astonished and said "I have never seen a patient's liver function return to normal this quickly. It's amazing."***

*Thank you again for sharing your expertise with seekers like myself—it's been life-changing so far. I look forward to deepening my practice. Peace.*

THOMAS COZZOLINO,
Technical Professional

# INTRODUCTION

People come to qigong for all kinds of reasons. Maybe you are seeking physical, mental, or emotional health. Perhaps you want to de-stress. Maybe you have trouble sleeping at night, and aches and pains call to you throughout the day. Perhaps you feel stuck in your life and your body is mirroring that back to you. Possibly you've tried different things—massage, yoga, or some traditional therapy years ago. Lately, the chiropractor just does not seem to be working.

You have heard about qigong; in fact, you might even have taken a Tai Chi class once.

There are more than three thousand styles of qigong practiced by more than eight million people every day in China alone.

What accounts for this popularity?

Qigong works! People are finding pain relief, stress relief, and exponential increases in their energy levels. Many even report total cures from supposedly incurable illnesses like stage four cancers.

## A Personal Healing Story

Whatever draws you to qigong (pronounced "chee gong"), I hope that qigong brings you all that it has brought me. I have used qigong as what I call a "power tool" to detoxify my mind and my body. I have used it to accelerate my own healing and well-being. To me it is a life hack, a shortcut.

After an accident in middle school in which a large trailer ran over my body on a farm, my life dramatically changed. By the time I was fifteen years old, I had been diagnosed with severe scoliosis and told that I would be crippled by the time I was thirty.

I was mentally, emotionally, and physically distraught. Although I was grateful that I had walked away from the accident, I was determined to undo all that it caused and more. I decided that my mind was more powerful than my body, but I knew this was an intellectual concept that I needed to somehow embody and subsequently demonstrate. I therefore became my first great experiment—I wanted to see if I could incorporate qigong into my life and use it as a means to heal my spinal disease and more.

In my mid-teens, I was introduced to qigong, medical qigong, and martial arts. Medical qigong is a primary form of medicine in China and it is considered the father of the more modern acupuncture. In acupuncture practice, a Doctor of Acupuncture inserts extremely thin needles into specific points along the body to impact the flow of energy or "chi" through the body. The medical qigong doctor or master (typically through many years of qigong and—often—martial arts practice) can sense blockages in a patient's energy pathways and/or the energy field that both surrounds and permeates the body. When medical qigong practitioners sense a blockage in one or more of the energy pathways or the field itself, they may use light touch, hot hands, sound, and other techniques to restore the chi flow.

In the years following that initial exposure I was introduced to Kenpo Karate, Kung Fu, Jeet Kune Do, Filipino martial arts, Aikido, Tae Kwon Do, and some other martial arts. I was astounded to see so many different yet complementary forms of qigong being practiced within these disciplines. I was also learning various forms of seated meditation and being exposed to an overall philosophy of connection to nature, to existence, to my deepest inner self. My search during those early years focused on healing myself—eliminating mental and physical pain and reducing daily emotional suffering. I had no intention of becoming a teacher of any of these disciplines.

In my late teens, I began studying Western psychology and emergency medicine at the University of Connecticut. I went on to study molecular and cellular biology at the University of Colorado and worked as a supervisor, team leader, and psychotherapist at a local hospital before going on to take classes for medical school.

Wherever I went, I brought my stress-reducing, pain-inhibiting, healing qigong practices with me. Whether I was at the hospital working or recovering from a full-contact karate tournament, I used my qigong practices to calm my mind, conserve my energy, and heal my body.

In my early twenties, people began seeking me out for healing. I had no sign, no business cards, and no website, but people were drawn to me and began asking me for help. I set up a treatment table at my house, and family and friends would come over and ask me to work on them. They would also ask me to teach them the practices so they could heal themselves, lose weight, get in shape, increase their energy, and stay healthy.

I would passionately share with them what I had learned and would also practice medical qigong treatments on those who lay on my treatment table. One by one, people were having amazing transformations. At that time I was still suffering with a spinal disease and the pain was often unbearable. Their healing experiences reinforced my belief and my hope that one day I would heal myself. When I was 25, I was seen by two physicians who, after looking at my x-rays, told me that—based on the condition of my spine—I would be crippled within five years. They told me that my spine looked like I was 85, it was arthritic, and I should prepare for the worst. According to the doctors, my spine would crush my lungs and internal organs and I would experience even greater pain and discomfort.

I had been doing qigong and martial arts for 10 years as well as receiving acupuncture, massage, chiropractic, and other forms of healing. I was deeply distressed, and had no idea what else I could possibly do.

I began working more deeply with my mind, my thoughts, and my emotions. I sought out master teachers and went more deeply into the practice of qigong and yogic breathwork called pranayama (which I now incorporate into my own style of qigong practice). I began an intensive breathing practice coupled with various qigong movements and still poses. I placed a significant emphasis on these particular practices over the course of about three years.

One day I was receiving a medical qigong treatment from a master practitioner and practicing healing breath during the session when energy surged through my body like a river. It was painful at first because I could feel this intense resistance keeping the energy from flowing, but then it turned incredibly blissful. I had several follow-up experiences like this, both during treatments and during my personal practice.

In so many ways, my body became enlivened and I experienced more space within myself. I was less agitated and my intuition had increased exponentially. It was not as if I was enlightened and all my troubles were over, but it was significant.

Then one day I was standing near a river with my shirt off, and my father shouted, "Your spine is straight!" Shortly thereafter I went to a doctor for a checkup, and the arthritis and scoliosis were gone!

I had noticed that I had not been in quite as much pain, had not been taking ibuprofen like candy recently and felt much freer on many levels. I had done the "impossible," and I knew I owed that to my qigong-breathing practices and the medical qigong treatments I received. In the days that followed, it became clear to me that my spine was totally healed.

A few years later, I had a full-time private practice treating people using medical qigong, offering mental, emotional, and physical counseling; medical intuition; and life coaching sessions. I also began teaching clients various qigong exercises to help them accomplish their health and life goals.

I often tell people that if I had to heal myself today, it would likely take three years or less, not thirteen. The science, techniques, and tools that I learned in those last three years caused a tipping point that I will never forget.

As a medical qigong practitioner, qigong teacher, and life coach, I am all about authentic shortcuts (life hacks) and I am all about results.

What qigong did for me was transformative! It changed me from the inside out and that changed my life in so many ways—it is quite incredible. Not only has qigong transformed my life, but I have taught thousands of people around the world through live workshops—in large part thanks to the Internet—to use qigong to heal themselves, increase their energy levels, facilitate healing for other people, increase their confidence and personal power, and become a channel for this universal life force called chi.

It is my intention that this information finds its way to people who are willing to make use of these concepts, ideas, philosophies, techniques, and teachings. At the beginning, you might dabble here and dabble there, and that is most appropriate. Once you see for yourself what it feels like to be qigong-high (no toxic side effects) and you see the results—increased physical energy, increased mental clarity, and improved personal and business relationships—I think you'll begin to appreciate the great benefits of this practice.

I was looking for a healing shortcut—I did not want to suffer so much pain and disease. Not every martial art or every form of qigong is going to work for every person. Not every book on positive thinking is going to help you change your most deep-seated beliefs and your views on reality. I am not here to tell you that my way is the only way and I am not here to tell you that all qigong practices will heal you; I personally think that some are much more potent than others. I base this only on personal experience of my own healing and on all of the healings I have helped facilitate through these practices.

I obviously believe that qigong practice is a big part of what I wish to share with you (hence the name of the book). Throughout this book, however, I will be sharing self-empowerment and self-healing tools I have learned along the way that I believe contribute to healing and the process of self-improvement. Some will be from Western psychology, some from Eastern psychology. I will share concepts that I have learned from many different master teachers, healers, shamans, and coaches. You will not necessarily know which style or which teacher or which perspective I'm drawing on for a particular teaching. Mostly, I'll be taking all of what I learned and conveying it in my own way.

Although I have been lucky enough to study with many masters, I really discovered how powerful qigong, martial arts, meditation, mindfulness practices, etc. are because I practiced them and eventually embodied them. That makes them mine. When you embody the teachings I share with you in this book, they will then be yours. You will carry them and share them as you choose to.

In my qigong teachings, I do offer a curriculum, because to master the basics and move forward in your life I think it is necessary. I also think that this book is an excellent adjunct to your study of qigong, although it's not a substitute for practice. If you like, you can learn and refine your practice using our online videos and, of course, our live seminars. My intent is for you to not only heal yourself, but to also serve others. I believe that service helps you heal yourself, other people, and the planet. That is why I certify qigong instructors and medical qigong practitioners—so that they can do what I have done, and be of service to others if they wish.

Bruce Lee, the famous movie star and martial artist, took the best attributes from each martial art he studied—and he studied many—and turned them into his own style of martial arts. Similarly, I have taken all of the best attributes that I have discovered from all of my teachers and all of my studies to create what you will see and learn in this book.

I believe that in order to heal yourself, you need to evolve to higher levels of awareness. This evolution of awareness comes from connection with yourself first and foremost. It cannot be achieved in someone else's way. It comes from self-discovery and self-empowerment, and qigong can be a useful tool for getting to know yourself deeply. At first you too might learn many techniques, concepts, and philosophies, but as you practice and integrate them into your life, you may go beyond what you have been taught to something even greater. You do not get there through dabbling, however, but through consistent effort.

I present qigong to you as a foundational practice that will allow you to tap into your own inherent greatness. Today more and more scientists are discovering the benefits of mind-body medicine, alternative medicine, traditional Chinese medicine, the power behind our thinking, the power of our words to influence biological processes, and so much more!

This is all very important, and yet it is only as good as your practice of some technique or exercise that allows you to become so proficient in changing your blood pressure (for example) that you can do it in a split second when you need it the most. Qigong is such a technique or exercise, and can help you learn to control bodily functions, pain, mood, etc.

A note of clarification—in the following chapters, you'll find two types of qigong activities: practices and exercises. Practices generally indicate qigong forms that don't require much physical exertion, and exercises involve more physical movements. Both are valuable and provide access to qigong for everyone, regardless of physical or other limitations.

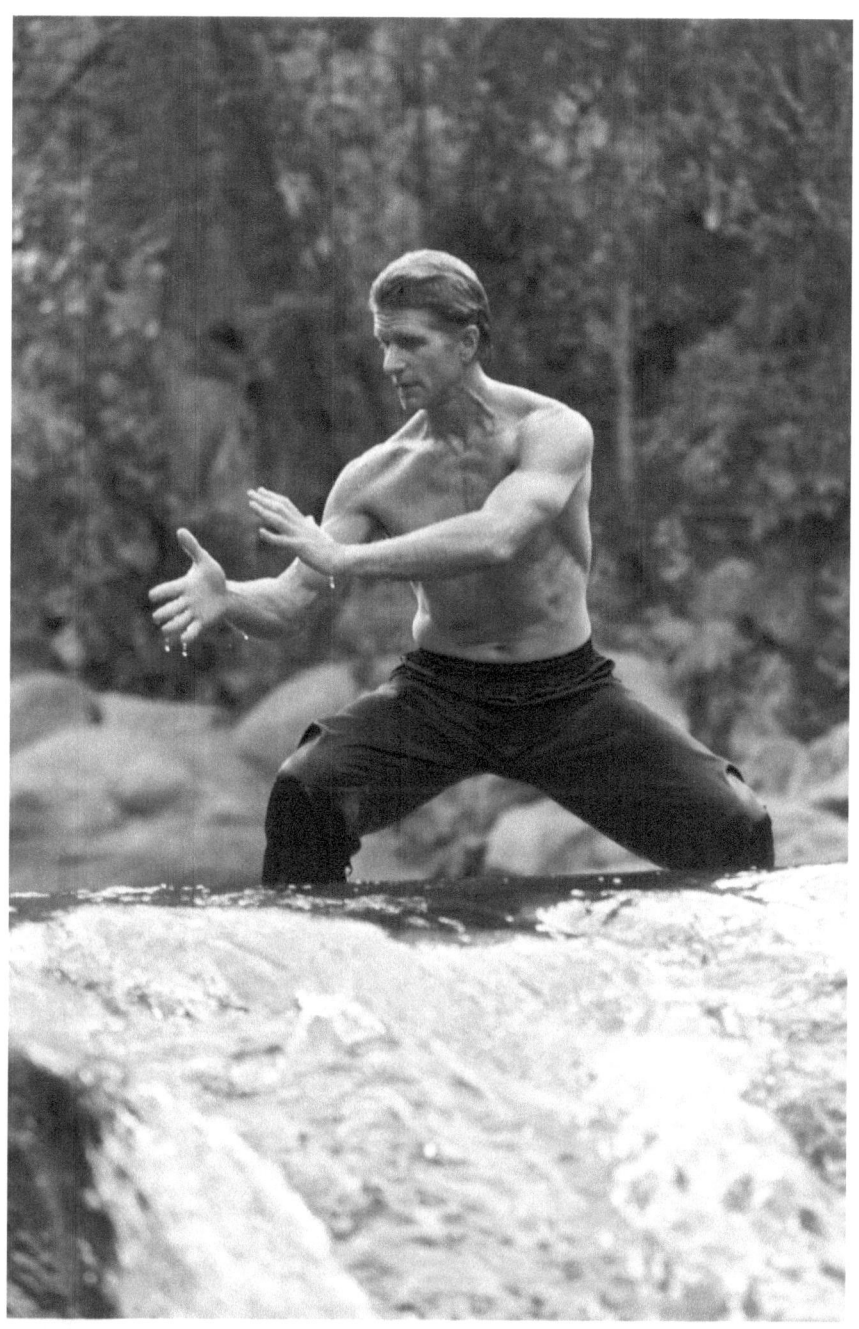

*Photo by: Lisa Siciliano*

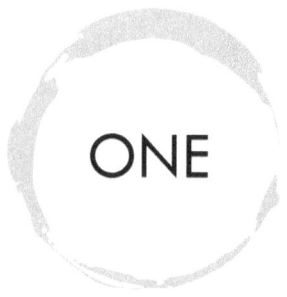

# ONE

# HOW DOES IT WORK?

"If you want to be healthy and live to one hundred years…
do qigong." Dr. Oz

Qigong can be translated as the skilled cultivation of the universal life force or "chi." Chi can be thought of as an electrical charge, a form of electromagnetism. All the body's inner workings operate through communications and instructions that involve electrical charge. You have little awareness of what is going on in your cells and their communications with each other, yet that process keeps you alive.

The human body is like a battery in that it has the ability to hold a charge. When you feel as if your battery is low and you are running on empty, you actually are. How do you recharge yourself and get that vital energy back? In Western terms, you might think of vitamins, supplements, and healthy foods. You might think in terms of fresh water and sunshine. All of these do contribute to your health, and it may also be helpful to think in terms of chi. Chi is considered in the Orient to be a universal life force energy. It is referred to as ki (pronounced "key") in Korea and Japan and it is referred to as prana in India.

Chi can be thought of as raw energy, and it runs in, around, and through your body. The most basic principle of Oriental medicine is that if chi is bountiful and flowing freely, then your body is strong, healthy, and vibrant; you have lots of energy; and—according to traditional teachings— you will be prosperous and live a long life. When the chi is stagnating, weak, or toxic, you develop sickness, lethargy, moodiness, aches and pains, etc. It is also said that if you and your body are stagnating and lethargic, your life must follow suit—where there is a lack of chi flow, there will also be a lack of opportunity and prosperity. As I will discuss later in the book, no energy, no passion; no passion, no power; no power, no ability to influence your life positively.

Qigong is the skilled practice of gathering more chi, more vital life force, more energy to yourself and harnessing and harmonizing it. Everything you do takes energy and actually either adds to your energy system or depletes it.

In traditional Chinese medicine, chi is a vast subject. For the purposes of this discussion, though, let's narrow the focus to chi essence or jing. In the Chinese language, jing means essence. According to traditional Chinese medicine and ancient Taoist texts, you receive a certain amount of this vital essence from your parents before you are born. This chi is called prenatal jing. Then whatever jing you have after being born is called post-natal jing.

This is briefly worth noting because whatever essence-energy you received from your parents you've got. For some it is a little and for some it is a lot. Either way, what is important for our purposes is that post-natal jing, which is the chi you have after you are born, can be built and developed! You can improve on your condition, whatever it is! Even in today's modern world of science, scientists have discovered that you can and do influence the expression of your genes. So even if you inherited less then healthy genes, you can alter their expression through, for example, exercise.

Whatever your state of chi, you can further develop it. Vitamins, herbs, and even good foods can only give you so much energy. If you are trying to take care of yourself and working with your diet and doing some exercise but the energy, the passion, the motivation is still not there or you feel like something is still missing, it could be that your chi is depleted.

Words like chi can seem strange because they come from a different culture and a different language, but hang in there. I will be speaking English throughout this book and it won't get any more complicated than what you just read. I am also going to ground this sometimes esoteric practice of qigong in basic science—science of breath, science related to the mind and brain, and so on.

Chi in its most pure form is raw and clean, free, and everywhere. It can simply be thought of as energy and it can also loosely be thought of as oxygen, although in traditional Chinese medicine and Taoist practice, chi is an invisible life force that is said to ride on the breath. Although it is everywhere, it requires skill to harness it. Water is also almost everywhere, but if you harness it and confine it in your own personal reservoir, you have a potential energy source at your disposal to generate more energy, fill your river, or help you grow your corn. That is power.

Greater qualities and quantities of chi (energy) are available to us through the skilled practice of qigong. Asian masters have demonstrated the profound power of qigong by performing seemingly impossible feats. Masters have bent spears with their throats saying that they used chi to protect themselves. Other masters have used their heads to break concrete blocks without even a scratch. Many masters have begun qigong practice to heal themselves of a childhood illness, an injury sustained during martial arts practice, or to recover from a war wound. Many masters and doctors of medical qigong have demonstrated incredible healing feats, dissolving cancerous tumors within a patient without even touching them.

As I mentioned, chi is said to ride on the breath and is delivered to our body's internal energy system and its cells, organs, and tissues by the breath. Not only is the blood charged by an influx of oxygen and the removal of carbon dioxide, but the blood is also charged as new chi enters on the breath.

So qigong practice places a huge emphasis on breathing, breath observation, and breath control. This is not the only way your body takes in and exchanges chi, though, because you—your body and your mind— are made up of electromagnetic fields, and these fields are energy fields. They are also chi fields.

If that seems like a preposterous idea, remember that the only reason electrocardiography (EKG) can measure heart activity is because a scientist discovered that the heart has an energy field and worked out how to measure it. Similarly, the only reason the electroencephalogram (EEG) can measure brain activity is because the brain emits a field of energy that can be measured. Yet when qigong masters talk about field therapy or the fact that they can sense certain things in these fields and influence them, it can sound bizarre. I am here to help bridge the gap between ancient science and modern medicine and give you enough information to make the practices more accessible.

The exhalation is designed to remove toxins from the body and its blood stream. Most of us have a very poor exhalation, however, because we unconsciously hold our breaths. This is why exercise is so important and why running, biking, and swimming improve your health and well-being. It is not simply that these exercises keep you slim and trim so that you can fit into your designer jeans—they also move and replenish your breath and therefore your chi, too. As you exercise harder, you breathe harder. As you breathe harder, you exhale today's stress and yesterday's poisons and this cleans your blood. Some people don't like to bike, swim, run, etc. Even if you do, you will have your down days. On the days when you are too tired or injured, qigong can fill the gap and keep you on track, expedite the healing process, and get you back in the game again.

If you don't like to exercise vigorously or if you are injured and cannot exercise vigorously, qigong is an excellent substitute and/or adjunct practice.

## Poor Breathing Habits

When a doctor tells you to "take a deep breath," he or she is doing a particular evaluation. As long as you are taking twelve to twenty breaths a minute and there are no signs of labored breathing, heart murmurs, etc., you are given a clean bill of health on that front. Even if you have perfect breathing from a Western medical perspective, you may still have anxiety, pain, digestive issues, etc.

A qigong doctor or master looks at and listens to your breath too. Sometimes with a stethoscope because Western medicine is also common in some Chinese hospitals, but often qigong masters listen without a stethoscope, and the breath can tell them a lot. It tells them how shallow your breath is, for example. If your breath is shallow, you most likely have symptoms like pain, allergies, tiredness, anxiety, etc.—all signs of poor breathing habits.

It can also tell a qigong master or doctor of medical qigong where you are breathing and where you are not breathing. Did you know that you are either breathing to your liver or you are avoiding breathing to your liver? Did you know that if your shoulder is in pain, you are holding your breath in that area and that this is blocking the chi and keeping the electrical impulses and blood and lymph from flowing through that area? So, someone skilled in this kind of listening can make some very important evaluations and help provide natural healing strategies for the situation.

It is possible, if you think it through logically, that cancer, for example, could be caused in part by poor breathing habits. Poor breathing habits can be due to stress and other forms of stagnation, including an injury to some area of the body. If more than 70% of all the toxins in your blood are supposed to be removed through exhalation but you are holding your breath, then toxins are not being successfully removed from your blood.

If that occurs, the lymphatic system can become backed up. If the lymphatic system becomes backed up, it becomes more likely that cancerous cells normally removed via the lymphatic system begin to build up and stagnate there. When cancer cell growth is then encouraged by sugar and reduced cell oxygenation, this sets the stage for the disease called cancer.

A healthy, vital, oxygenated body can better keep cancer in check, but when the body becomes overtaxed and under-oxygenated, cancer is given an extra advantage and can become very problematic. Remember that chi is said to ride on the breath and specifically even upon the oxygen itself. Whether we see energy in terms of chi or electromagnetic energy or fields of energy, oxygenation versus lack of oxygenation is of the utmost importance to our health. Oxygenation leads to health, lack of oxygen leads to both aging and disease.

Regardless of what condition you have, be it scoliosis and extreme back pain like I did, or cancer or lethargy or fatigue or anxiety or depression or some other form of discomfort, we really need to detoxify the blood if we want to improve our mental, emotional, and physical states of health and well-being. There are various things you can do to detoxify the blood, but—first and foremost—you would be wise to detoxify your breath through conscious exhalation followed by conscious inhalation.

Although this is absolutely true, I do not believe that this will ever be enough, in and of itself, to completely heal your body and radically improve your life. It is, however, a key ingredient. Conscious and purposeful breathing is only one aspect of the qigong practices that I will teach you, yet it is an important component of these exercises and one to absolutely make note of.

Also, when someone asks you, "How does qigong contribute to your health?" you can answer them by saying, "Well, do you realize that many of the toxins in your blood are removed through your exhalation? And did you realize that most of us are holding that exhalation and holding our breath in? Qigong really works with our breathing and this helps us detoxify our blood."

In order to truly take a deep breath, you need to first work on the exhalation; you need to work on getting the bad breath out. Once you create space by removing the old breath with its carbon dioxide and other wastes, you will begin to breathe new oxygen, new chi (which rides on the oxygen) into your lungs, into your belly and into your blood. When blood becomes old, stagnant, undernourished and under-oxygenated, it loses its vitality and it literally causes you pain. The cells in your tissues are under-oxygenated, and this creates the buildup of a poison called lactic acid. The body produces lactic acid when there is not enough oxygen for the cells. Lactic acid building up in the muscles and playing upon the nerves causes pain.

## Athletes Build Up Lactic Acid

Athletes know this well, and when they keep running and do not have enough oxygen to keep them going, the body shifts into an anaerobic form of energy production that creates lactic acid. This lactic acid causes muscles and tissues to tighten up and hurt.

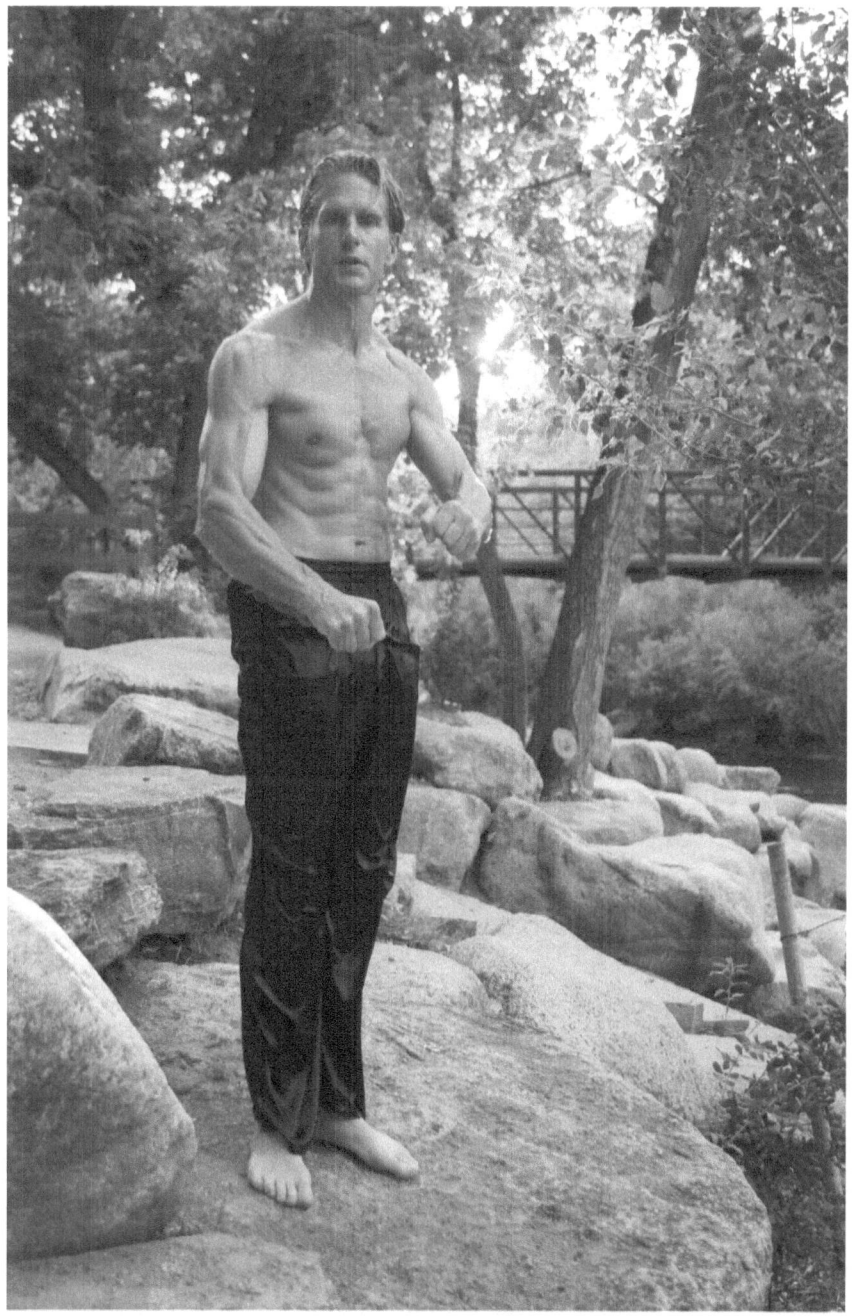

*Photo by: Lisa Siciliano*

If you do not exercise strenuously and/or are not very healthy, you are likely experiencing the same problem. Poor breathing habits lead to a form of energy production that happens when you aren't taking in enough oxygen. The body will keep producing energy for you, breaking down the food you eat into the body's main source of energy (from a Western science, nutritional, and biological perspective), a molecule called adenosine triphosphate. This comes at a price—lactic acid. The tightness and pain this causes further inhibits you from taking a deep breath. This begins to create a vicious cycle that—if not addressed—can lead to more and more health problems.

Because chi rides on the breath and that invisible breath feeds a massive matrix of chi pathways and electrical neural nets, conscious breathing practices are of the utmost importance. Breathing deeply and correctly can detoxify the blood and can eventually lead to control over emotions and mental processes. This helps prevent stress and further toxicity in the blood and in all cellular functions.

If you also have the wisdom to understand that the internal hardware is all electrical hardwiring, then you would be wise enough to know that this is going to emit an electromagnetic field and that all electromagnetic fields attract and repel other electromagnetic fields. So your electrical hardwiring makes you an energy field. That field is electromagnetic. This makes you like a walking magnet.

Electromagnetic fields may sound a little woo-woo, but Western science has known about some of these fields for some time now. As I mentioned, Western medicine regularly uses technology that measures both the field given off by your heart and the field given off by your brain. Tests like the EKG would not be possible without the scientific discovery of these fields.

That also means that your collective energy field, your personal magnetism, is attracting other people's energy fields as well as repelling them. So your best self defense is not necessarily the most lethal martial art—it is a clean mind, clean body, clean emotional state, and clean circuitry, because magnets of like energy attract each other! When it comes to electromagnetic fields, like attracts like. The policeman attracts the bad guy, the doctor attracts the sick guy, the qigong master attracts the student who wants to heal. It is not exactly that simple, but it's a useful way to begin to think about it.

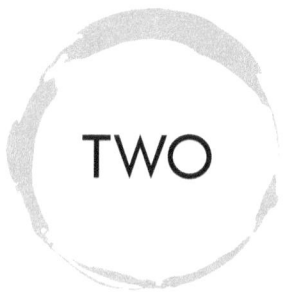

# TWO

# HARNESSING YOUR ENERGY

"People always ask me when they see me working out, "What are you training for?" The answer is I'm training for life." Laird Hamilton

When we practice qigong, we use a particular mindset, a focused, yet relaxed, mind. This takes time to understand, but it helps to have that as a goal right from the start. Where your mind goes, chi flows. As your mind begins to direct energy, whether it is through your breath or controlling your temperature or your blood pressure, where your mind goes the energy will go, the heat will go, and your body will respond accordingly. This takes practice—you cannot do these types of things just because you comprehend them intellectually. Practice is essential; for example, you can rely on skilled breathing techniques in a stressful moment when you need them the most only if you have practiced them one hundred times in the comfort of your home under less stressful conditions.

Imagine taking a physical qigong posture and standing with your knees slightly bent and legs just past the shoulders, as if you were riding a horse. Then imagine placing your hands over your lower belly just below the navel center with one hand right on top of the other. Imagine yourself holding this pose and, when you are ready, stand and assume the pose. If you are already familiar with this exercise, read on to add some philosophy and theory to your practice and see if you can improve it.

As you assume this posture, you are not only stepping into a qigong pose that has been practiced for more than five thousand years, but you are also placing your hands on what is referred to in Oriental medicine and qigong practice as the lower dantian. This is a major shortcut, a gift given to us by masters who have gone before us.

If you practice qigong long enough and have enough success with it, you will discover this area also referred to in Japanese martial arts as the hara. You would discover that it is a center of heat, a center of chi, a center of kundalini fire, and a center of personal power. This area of the navel center is also referenced in yogic practices as housing what yogis call the nadis egg. It is a central energy hub from which some 350 million energy channels associated with 350 million nerves are said to run.

Because someone was kind enough to pass the information along to me, and I'm passing it along to you, you can take advantage of this shortcut of placing your attention on the lower dantian. You might have discovered it on your own after ten thousand hours of meditation, but most Westerners are unlikely to meditate for 10,000 hours—or even five hours—unless they are told why it is worth the effort and how it will benefit them. So I am here to offer you the why and the how. The doing is up to you, although I will coach you through that too if you would like my assistance.

After practicing qigong and martial arts for more than thirty years, when I send healing energy to some part of my body or to a client or patient, I am very aware of my lower dantian as a source of my heat, internal energy, and internal power. When I punch or kick or break a concrete block with my hand, I am aware of this area of my body and inner being as a source of power.

In the fitness industry, it is becoming common knowledge that we must engage our core on a regular basis to have more overall strength, flexibility, and power. This is old news for qigong and martial arts practitioners. The core (the abdomen) has always been seen as an essential part of practices associated with qigong, health, and vitality.

The fitness world also emphasizes the strength of the stomach muscles, which may be important depending on what you do. Underneath the skin and muscle, though, there is an important reservoir for internal power that is either filled with energy or has become depleted of it. This energy source, this core, is closely associated with the organs in your body and your organs play a big role in the health and vitality of your tissues. If you have soreness in your tissues—the back of your neck or your shoulders, for example—chances are you have an issue of stagnation in one or more of your organs.

## Qigong Postures

When you sit or stand in any posture, you are affecting the mind and the mind's mental posture (position of the self and the environment of people, places, and things surrounding the self), your emotions, and the various energetic fields. You are either contributing to the flow of chi or you are causing chi to stagnate. You may not realize yet the power of a posture, so imagine something opposite to a qigong practice such as standing hunched over for half an hour. If you were healthy and you stood hunched over for a half an hour and occasionally made a coughing sound, you would make yourself sick.

The opposite, of course, is also true, and this exemplifies how qigong practice works. If you were stressed or sick or both and you stood in this qigong pose as if you were riding a horse and you bring your hands to the lower dantian and you stand there still, you begin to harness your chi. You begin to organize the chi that flows around you very differently compared to how the chi would flow if you were to hunch over.

Remember that where your mind goes, your chi flows. So when you place your hands at the lower belly just below the navel center, you are focusing on the area that houses this epicenter of energy. The problem for most people is that the tank is mostly empty.

To develop a greater awareness of what is there and what can be built there, we need to begin to put our attention there. As we do, little by little, the energy will build there. There are, of course, techniques that will get you there more slowly and there are techniques that take you there more quickly. Most disciplines require that you learn to walk before you learn to run, so you can choose your favorite practices accordingly.

## Attention and Ancient Alchemy

Wherever you place your hands, you are focusing your attention. Your attention is potent! Very potent! The more attention you have, the more you will cultivate energy and the more energy you cultivate, the more energy you will be able to direct. So you must practice harnessing your attention—you must master holding your own attention to be successful in anything you do.

You can direct your attention and energy for personal healing purposes or you can direct your attention and energy to improve your healing technique in acupuncture or massage. The ability to direct your attention and energy is also useful in martial arts and will help you stay grounded and in your power center during a business negotiation or a confrontation with an assailant. You can use your built-up chi to have great sex, build a great business, leave everyone in your dust running up that mountain this weekend, heal a physical injury, have a baby, or stay up late with the two you already have.

The lower belly (dantian) is like a bank account that houses energy and heat. How much you have in your account determines how much you have to spend, save, or invest. Without this essential energy in the lower belly, though, your sexual energy, your vitality, your longevity, and your kidneys and their vitality are all compromised. From a traditional Chinese medicine and Taoist perspective, everything else is either built up from there or depleted from there. Some male competitors in the jiu jitsu world, such as the infamous Rickson Gracie, know the benefits of not having sex prior to competition. I believe Rickson does not have sex for two weeks prior to a fight. He also eats very healthily prior to his bouts. Rickson Gracie has been undefeated in more than five hundred competitions, including mixed martial arts competitions, with competitors from around the world.

The lower dantian is associated with your sexual organs, your sexual energy, and your primary source of vitality. Your kidneys are also primary organs associated with this area of your body, and they are a primary giver or taker of your vital life force. If the lower dantian is weak and depleted of energy, so are your kidneys, so are you, and—most likely—so is your sex life. As you'll see throughout this book, building up the lower dantian is an extremely important part of your road to healing and self-improvement.

As you hold your hands over the lower belly and stand in this posture of meditation, you begin to gather subtle energy to yourself. Moments ago that energy was being scattered all over your world, wherever your mind was going off to, but now you are starting to call it back to your center, to your core. In time, this will begin to develop a heat in the dantian. It will rebuild lost energy stores and rebuild sexual energy (essential energy that can be, but does not have to be, expressed sexually). It will also further build that energy if you are mindful and consistent, and, as it does, the heat that develops in the belly will rise to the solar plexus and eventually all the way to the top of the head. We will discuss this in more detail later.

As I mentioned, the lower dantian, known as the hara in some Japanese martial arts like Aikido, is considered a place of power. It is also seen in many meditative practices as a cauldron or melting pot. It is the pot, the crucible, in which the qigong practitioner alchemizes metaphorical lead into metaphorical gold.

In ancient times, practitioners of qigong were referred to as alchemists (see CHAPTER FIVE: THE ALCHEMIST).

These ancient qigong practitioners would take the lead, the heaviness, the stress of the past, the emotional memories, the body memory, the anger, the sadness, the greed, the jealousy, the pain, etc., and burn the energy that held those emotions in the lower belly until the energy began to rise, purging and detoxifying the body and cleansing the mind. The practitioner then became like a phoenix, the mystical bird that rises from its own ashes purified and reborn.

This alchemical process is sometimes referred to as ascension, hinted at in the caduceus, a Western medicine symbol. In this symbol, which you see at hospitals, in doctors' offices, and on doctors' business cards, there are two snakes that wrap around a staff. The snakes meet at the top of the staff and the two heads come together. This does not belong only to Western medicine—it is a symbol that can be found in many ancient teachings.

This symbol represents kundalini, which is a concentrated chi (energy) that is said to be coiled up at the base of the spine like a snake. It lies there dormant waiting to be activated. When it is activated through qigong practice, kundalini yoga, medical qigong treatments, or certain forms of deep meditation, it rises. Not only does the energy itself rise through the snakes (called ida and pingala in yogic philosophy), it rises through the staff called shushumna in yogic sciences as well. Some say that shushumna is the same energy pathway that is referenced in traditional Chinese medicine and Taoist practices such as Chong Mai.

When opened and flooded with energy, these pathways can lead to deep healing, experiences of non-duality, and the evolution of mood and conscious awareness. These pathways are also said to activate the endocrine system and hormones (cell-to-cell communicators), boost immunity, reverse aging, and so much more.

## Qigong, Yogic Philosophy, and the Endocrine System

It is also interesting to note the relationship between the seven chakras in Indian medicine, which are seen as major vortices of energy, and our endocrine systems. These major energy centers—one at the base of the spine, one at the navel center, one at the solar plexus, one at the heart, one at the throat, one at the third eye, and one at the crown—are all associated with major endocrine glands. This indicates that the endocrine system and the chakras, which are whirling vortices of energy, are intimately related and are a major source of internal and external health.

## Oriental Medicine, Jing, and True Heat

When you sit quietly in Buddha pose or you stand quietly in a qigong pose and hold your hands over the lower belly, just below the navel center, you begin to activate your cauldron, your lower dantian. When that begins to generate heat, the heat will rise and spread over and throughout the body. In Oriental medicine, this is sometimes referred to as true heat.

Also, note that the lower belly is considered our core, and when it is cold outside, our extremities like fingers, toes, nose, and ears are the first to get cold. The reason for this is that our core contains our organs and the body considers these organs to be more important than toes and fingers. So the heat is kept so that the organs can stay nice and warm. And unless the core is warm enough, the belly will not share its warmth.

This idea occurs often in qigong and Oriental medicine. Unless the core has enough jing, enough fire (true heat or ming-men, which is associated with the kidneys), it will not share it with the rest of the body. So if someone has weakened chi, regardless of the specific symptoms, you can be sure the lower belly does not have enough chi, enough jing, enough potency, or true fire (ming-men).

So if your chi is weak, your energy low, and your passion deflated, you'll want to increase heat in the basement of your belly. Any practice that accomplishes that will allow you to begin developing greater vitality.

## A Special Note for Healing Practitioners

If a client has depleted chi, be sure to incorporate concentrated chi transmissions to their lower dantian in order to increase the chi there. You can further activate the area of the ming-men fire that is directly associated with the kidneys. Those of you who are acupuncturists know the ming-men acupuncture point and can use that as a direct point of chi transmission.

This can also be done by laying both hands just under your client's belly button as you stand in a qigong pose as if you are sitting on a horse. With your hands on your client's belly, hold the area, observe, relax, watch your breath, let the energy build in your own belly, and allow some of it to pass to your client. Another way to offer a client or fellow practitioner a chi boost is to hold their ankles, place your fingers along or near the kidney meridian, and visualize sending energy up both legs to the kidneys.

## Signs of Developing Chi

Whether you are practicing qigong for yourself or observing and assisting someone else through medical qigong transmission, there are a few signs to look for. These include heat building in the hands and belly and warmth running through the core and spreading up the body and out to the extremities.

Also be alert for subtle swallows that come all on their own and for those swallows to turn into deeper breaths that happen automatically. You may also notice the breath getting deeper and the ribs expanding all on their own. If you are working and practicing with yourself, this should be obvious, although it may take time to build up enough chi to impact your throat, your swallowing, and the endocrine juices in that swallow. If you are practicing medical qigong with someone else and offering them a healing, watch for these signs as well.

## Detoxifying Your Blood

Your blood is extremely important for your health and vitality, your energy stores, and your emotional state. For most people, toxins are not removed very effectively and their blood becomes loaded with various forms of toxicity.

Proper exhalation can remove many of the toxins in your blood. Stress, however, has become a problem of epic proportions, and stress causes you to hold your breath. Holding your breath can result in fear, feelings of separation, and—physically—disease.

Could so many of us holding our breath contribute to the state of human consciousness and the impact of that consciousness on the planet at large? You bet!

In ancient times, the breath and the spirit were synonymous. What is the first thing a baby does when it is born? It takes a deep breath. What is the last thing a body does as the spirit departs? There is an exhale without the follow-up of an inhale. Spirit and breath are related, and if you breathe deeply you bring your spirit into your body more fully. Similarly, when you hold your breath, you prevent your greater consciousness, your greater awareness, and the energy that surrounds you from replenishing you.

Breathing more deeply is a simple and effective strategy for improving your health, vitality, and perhaps even your life circumstances. Many people say they accept the support of existence or they are open to receive good things in their life. Many of those same people hold their breath. You can live without food for a couple of weeks and live without water for at least a few days, but most people cannot live without breath for more than several minutes.

Why do people hold their breath? Stress, right? Guarding, constriction, self-defense, fear, etc. This happens naturally for most people. If you saw a basketball coming at you and you had time to react, you might contract your body and hold your breath as you took the hit from the basketball. Martial artists train themselves to forcefully exhale their breath when they get hit with a punch or a kick, and they make a yelling sound. This sound forces air out and can protect the body from a blow or a strike. If you get a punch to the stomach and you happen to be either a) pausing in mid-breath or b) taking an in-breath, you will feel a tremendous amount of pain and nausea.

Holding the breath and staying in a state of contraction on a regular basis (which I would suggest most people are doing) is not at all good for you on many, many levels. When you hold your breath while eating as if you are in a race, without really relaxing and taking the time to breathe, you create a pressure in your belly and your body.

Have you ever heard a mother say "Johnny, stop inhaling your food"? She is wise to suggest this to her son, because a lack of mindfulness while eating means a lack of awareness of self and a subsequent lack of awareness of breathing. If you do not take the time to breathe between chewing and swallowing your food, you are creating a stressful internal situation. This type of eating contributes to emotional swelling and, subsequently, physical swelling, and for a lot of people this way of eating leads to excess weight gain.

Weight loss is not just about what you eat—it is also about how you eat. A meatball sandwich may not be the healthiest thing to eat but imagine someone eating a meatball sandwich very fast because they are in a hurry to get back to their job. Then imagine them racing through traffic because they are late. This wreaks havoc on the body. Although food consumption absolutely plays a role in optimum health, breath or the lack thereof also plays an important role in what you consume, how you consume it, and the effect it has on your body.

Once you consume your food, it will create toxins and many of those will end up in the blood. A great way to cleanse the blood is to practice exhaling, followed by deeper and deeper inhalations. Breathe out the toxins, breathe in new oxygen. Breathe in the raw energy of existence. Get rid of the toxic carbon dioxide. Get out the old, used, and stagnant breath and breathe in new vital life force.

The form of qigong I teach emphasizes the exhalation. It's an effective strategy to rid yourself of toxic, old, carbon dioxide-filled breath, and make room for new breath, new oxygen, and new chi.

Chi—energy, vital life force—rides on the breath. It comes in on the inhalation. You can then practice storing it and housing it in the lower belly. First, though, you must make room for new breath, new oxygen molecules, and new chi.

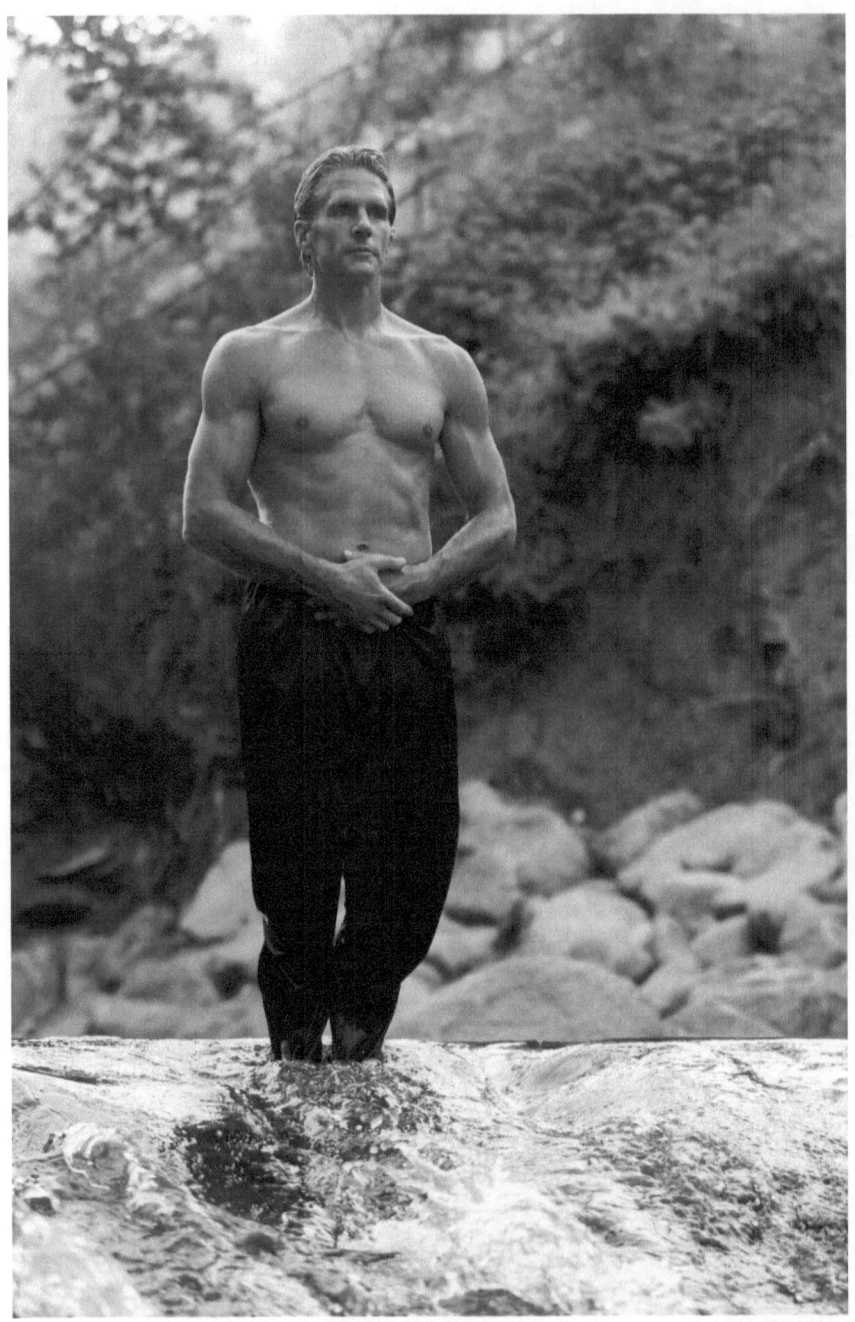

*Photo by: Lisa Siciliano*

## *Qigong Exercise: Detoxify Your Blood and Store Energy in Your Belly*

Here's how to detox your blood and create more space for more energy and more power in the belly:

- Take a slow deep breath in through your nose and raise your belly. Stress, anxiety, pain, etc. are produced when you breathe to your lungs and not your belly.
- After you take that breath into the lower belly, exhale that breath out and contract your belly a bit, then push that last bit of breath out. Repeat this exercise right now 5–10 times.
- Right now! Don't read on, do this simple practice first—it will only take one minute!
- I once read in a biology book that 70% of the toxins in your blood are cleaned up through your exhalation. I have taught this for many years since then. It is interesting that I cannot find the science on that anywhere. I cannot help but wonder why that is. Regardless, we know that carbon dioxide is poisonous and oxygen is essential. So practicing this type of exercise five, ten, or even better one hundred times will have an exponential healing effect in that it will oxygenate your cells. It will also change your mood and influence your energy levels. Don't take my word for it, do it!
- Know that with every exhale, you are helping your blood to detox and you are giving yourself room for new oxygen, new energy, new fuel, and new power.

Have you ever seen a Kung Fu master break a brick with his head, or be hit by a baseball bat at 90 mph, and the baseball bat breaks, but the master is unharmed? If not, check it out on YouTube. There is great energy and power in these practices. Even if you have no interest in learning practices like these, there is clearly something to these practices if a master of this type of practice can perform a superhuman feat like that!

Learning to control your breath generates great power. This power can be used to heal yourself and improve your focus. Understanding the practice more deeply can calm your nerves in the moments when you need your wits about you the most.

If you really want to cleanse your blood and your breath, try fasting with only lemon water for the day while practicing your breathing and qigong techniques to increase their effectiveness.

## Healing Benefits of This Exercise

This exercise can result in cleaner blood, cleaner tissues, less pain and inflammation, greater healing, stronger immune function, and more. Your blood is your life force. It carries oxygen and chi through your body. If it is toxic, you have problems. Cleaner blood means a cleaner bill of health! Simultaneously, you are making more space in the belly by getting rid of carbon dioxide and other poisons. This creates more room for new breath, more oxygen, and more energy.

## Qigong Exercise: Shortcut to Cleaner Blood

Stand as if you are sitting on a horse. Focus on the ground. Sink in a bit.

The closer your legs are to being under your shoulders, the easier it will be. The wider they are, the harder it will be. Discover what works best for you. Now inhale slowly through your nose, raising your hands up to the sky. Then let your arms and hands slowly come down in front of you, palms down toward the floor, falling slowly toward your waist as your breath comes out. When you get to the belly, roll your hands out away from you as if you are shooing away the bad energy from your belly. Meanwhile make the sound "ahhh," like you do at the doctor's when they ask you to open your mouth and say "ah." Let your exhalation out completely and then try to go past the normal exhalation and push out a little bit more. Do not strain! Then slowly inhale again.

Repeat this exercise five times.

To see this exercise on video and for more exercises like this to detoxify the blood and reduce inflammation in the body, check out my videos on Amazon: Qigong for Beginners and Qigong Challenge.

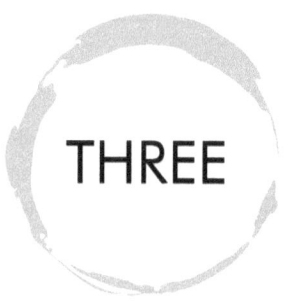

# THREE

# ENERGY EQUALS POWER

"One reason so few of us achieve what we truly want is that we never direct our focus; we never concentrate our power. Most people dabble their way through life, never deciding to master anything in particular." Tony Robbins

Everything you do either increases or diminishes your energy reserves. Everything you think, everything you do to others, everything you feel about yourself, everything you put in your body, everything you speak out loud—everything you do. Everything you do not do also increases or diminishes your energy system.

When I speak about your energy system, I am talking about this on a much more complex scale than simply whether or not you have enough energy to get out of bed in the morning. I am talking about that too, though!

I am talking about your passion, your drive, your sexual vitality, your excitement, your enthusiasm, your happiness, or your lack of some or all of those things. This place called Earth is a place of duality—light versus dark, happy versus sad, up versus down. Everybody is going to experience ups and everybody is going to experience downs. Rich people will, happy people will, sad people will.

Life around you will constantly change, but that does not have to be a bad thing. Nor does that have to be something that regularly drains your energy system. With some skill, you can harness and replenish your energy even during the challenging times. You will need all of your energy to influence your inner and outer world, especially during those times.

Energy is defined in physics as the ability to do work. If you consider yourself to be an alchemist (like I consider myself), then define your personal energy as your ability to do great works and turn lead into gold. If you are in any way unhealed, excessively suffering, overly confused, still carrying pain, illness, and disease, how many great works can you do? It is hard enough to get out of bed in the morning, right? My head hurts too much to make love; I have so little energy—how could I start my own business or expand the business I have? People say things like "I would heal this disease if it had not drained me of all of my energy. I just don't have what it takes anymore to continue."

But maybe things were going great for you right up until you injured yourself in your favorite sport or hobby. After that injury and even after physical therapy, etc., you cannot get back on top of your game. You may think that your "bad" attitude is due to your physical condition. I hear people say this kind of thing all the time, "I would be great if it weren't for my back." Or "Things would be great if I just was not in pain all the time. I just want to get back to running, weight lifting, or swimming, etc." I understand.

If you want to heal yourself regardless of your current circumstances, you'll need to cultivate subtle energy, life force. You'll need that fuel to help you get through any obstacle that arises, whether it is a personal relationship, a business issue, or a physical ailment or injury. Many people have to face several things at once. Where is the energy coming from that allows you to cope? Starbucks is not going to cut it here, especially if you can drink one or two cups of coffee and go to sleep. You following me?

Great news! You have access to far more energy than you realize! You have to eat right. You would be wise to eat organic greens and organic vegetables and sprouts. When you eat whole, organic food, your body and its cells will be happier and healthier. You may also want to take a few key vitamins like vitamin C, and if you are brave try some spirulina mixed into a glass of water or add to your favorite smoothie. Occasional fasting with just lemon water for the day will give your body and its organs a rest. And be sure to exercise. If you are already doing all of that to some degree, awesome!

It's still a good idea to add these qigong practices to your life, whether you have a good diet or not. The subtle energy that comes from your breath, your thoughts, and your declarations about your body and your life absolutely influences your personal reality, which includes you and all that you attract into your life.

No matter what you do in life, it requires energy. No energy, no passion; no passion, no desire; no desire and you become like a robot that doesn't care about itself or its environment. So if you want to improve your life and your circumstances then you need to gather some energy—get some stuff accomplished in the direction you truly desire to head and take your power back!

In physics, power is defined as the rate of doing work. In other words, how much power you have determines how much work gets done. Synonyms for power include ability, potential, capacity and competence. So healing, changing, or influencing your life requires energy and power. If you have little to no energy, you cannot possibly be powerful in anything you do.

When you think about personal energy, think also about personal power; the two go hand in hand. As you increase your personal energy stores, you will increase your personal power. Power can be thought of as the ability to act or do something in a particular way, including influencing the behavior of others. There is a big difference between having power over others and using your power to empower other people. I recommend the latter.

In this work, I encourage you to think about great power. I want you to think in terms of great energy, great power, and great works! If you can build up a reservoir of new energy stores, passion, drive, and enthusiasm, you will have more than some "thing" to give. You are going to have the energy and power to heal yourself and to change the circumstances of your life. If you begin to do that, you will automatically begin to positively influence those around you.

Whether your intent is to heal your body of some ailment or to change the outer circumstances of your life, you are going to require a lot of energy. Ever heard that before? Most people want to transform several things in their life not just one. People who have health challenges tend to have financial, relationship, career, or other challenges too. Energy is required to make changes in any one of those areas, because each area is reflecting inner challenges—bridges that must be crossed, walls that must be overcome!

The good news is all your challenges represent only one challenge. If you achieve positive change at the core of your being, you will positively influence your outer environment in a myriad of ways.

I also recommend that you look at your life more like a long distance race than a sprint, regardless of how old you are. From this perspective, I recommend you entertain longevity, and with longevity comes the potential for health, prosperity, and great works. No longevity and you just have a steady decline. Do not think in terms of hours and days; think in terms of months and years when it comes to making significant changes in your life. Tomorrow will always be here sooner than you think. If you don't make the effort today to improve yourself and your circumstances, you will need to rely on luck. Luck is great, but don't count on it to do all the work! You would be better off developing the habit of daily qigong practice.

## Qigong Exercise: Horse Stance and Holding the Lower Belly/Dantian

Whether you are facing physical health challenges and/or other life challenges, you will likely benefit from this practice. Energy is all around you—it is above you, below you, to the sides of you, surrounding you. But you have to harness it to use it.

Think about water that is left to dissipate. How powerful is it?

On the other hand, a reservoir filled with water has a great deal of potential energy. If you released water from the reservoir, you would see an awesome wave with dramatic effects. You need to learn to build up your own reservoirs if you want to be full of energy and raw power. High quality energy and raw power cannot be found in a soda can but you can "drink it" through your breath and through the ancient, internal practices of this style of qigong.

I recommend that you practice this next exercise every morning, afternoon, or evening for a week or two. Pick a time of day that works for you and be consistent.

- Stand with your knees slightly bent and legs just past the shoulders, as if you are riding a horse.
- Lay your hands just below your navel center. Hold your hands there and be still. Where your mind goes, energy will follow. It takes the mind to place the hands there and, after placing your hands there, your mind will begin to be present right there. More and more, every minute you hold your hands there, your mind follows and so does energy. Try this practice for five to eight minutes.
- What did you feel? Any warmth? Any tingling sensations in the body? Any swallows to the throat?
- Your lower belly is a special area of your body, a central core. It is the body's furnace. In alchemical practices of qigong, it is referred to as a cauldron. In Chinese medicine, it is referred to as the lower dantian. It is where you take metaphorical lead and turn it into metaphorical gold. The lead can be likened to your heavy emotions. These emotions and their reactions can either drain you or fuel you. If you become skilled at holding your hands to the lower belly for extended periods of time, (while seated or standing) you will begin to harness precious energy and develop internal power.
- This precious epicenter of your health and well-being has largely been forgotten. Forget about it and you are forgotten, because you are depleted in many more ways than you are currently aware of. So bring your awareness back to your center. Remember—where your mind goes, energy goes. For most people, energy has been going out in many different directions and therefore bringing back many mixed experiences. Before you try to bring about changes in your outer world, it is wise to bring your attention and your

awareness back to yourself and your physical center in the lower belly.

- Martial arts masters refer to this lower belly as the hara. All the martial arts masters I have ever met and trained with have talked about this area as the epicenter of their power. Whether they were a "soft style master" like a Tai Chi master or a "hard style master" like a Karate master, they always reference this area of the body.
- Taoist masters and masters of sexual Kung Fu associate this area with the kidneys, sexual energy, vital life force, and longevity.
- When was the last time you even noticed your belly, unless you were hungry or too full? Overall, the deeper teachings and functions of these practices regarding the lower dantian have been a well-kept and guarded secret for many centuries. They became public knowledge some forty years ago when a high Chinese official was healed of a terminal illness through qigong. That official made qigong available in many Chinese hospitals. Since then, word has spread. According to some sources, more than eight million people practice qigong in China on a daily basis.

As you hold this area of your body, you are charging the basement, the source of fire, of energy, and of passion. This area of the body is associated with sexual energy and desire, passion in general, and the kidneys, organs of longevity. No fire in the basement, not enough sexual energy; no fire in the basement, dysfunctional sexual energy. No fire in the basement, no drive; no drive, no passion; no passion, no healing energy. No internal power. No internal power, no external power to change your life for the better.

Try placing your hands on your lower belly for seven minutes every day for the next seven days. Just pick a time of day and do it!

- I dare you! Seven minutes a day for seven days, then report back.
- I double triple dare you!
- Do it! What do you have to lose?
- Hold that belly!

## *Healing Benefits of This Exercise*

Practiced diligently, this exercise can improve digestion, increase energy flow, regulate temperature, regulate blood pressure, energize the kidneys, increase libido, boost immune function, help manage pain, and quiet allergies and lung conditions. It also increases personal power and self-confidence and can increase fertility for both men and women.

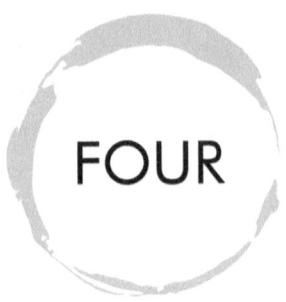

# FOUR

## HEALING

"Find out for yourself what are the possessions and ideals that you do not desire. By knowing what you do not want, by elimination, you will unburden the mind, and only then will it understand the essential which is ever there."
Jiddu Krishnamurti

When I speak of healing, I am speaking about mental, emotional, physical, and spiritual healing. This kind of healing is multidimensional, and each level is intimately intertwined with your life, your job, your family, and your career—all of it. Success is relative, and like everything else, it depends how you define it. You can be successful financially but have issues with alcoholism, stress, and dysfunctional relationships. You can be broke and have a happy, fulfilled life with less money. Some people are rich inside and out. You choose your state of health—or not—every day.

There has to be something better than surface-level success and surface-level failure, though, and there is. Have you ever heard the teaching, "Seek not outside yourself"? If I were to continue that statement, I would say,

"Seek not outside yourself for the source of your problems," and "Seek not outside yourself for the solution to your problems."

You are the source of your limitations and your pain, but you are also your greatest solution! Many people seek success outside themselves first and figure, "I will get around to inner success one of these days when I have more time, more money, and more energy." There's no time like the present, however, to take action and change the circumstances of your life.

## Multidimensional Healing

Multidimensional healing is challenging work. Most people who attempt healing approach it from one level, such as the physical. They will try to eat right and take their medicines and vitamins, maybe giving the rest to God or fate.

There is a lot more to healing than that, though. You are a thinker; a feeler; and a physically embodied being who can love, hate, create, preserve, and/or destroy. You have mental tapes that have run through your head from childhood, you have muscle memory from all the fight or flight reactions you have experienced, and you have complex neural nets that your thinking runs up, down, and along.

Your reality and your future are predetermined through your nervous system and your DNA. Unless you do something to change your hardwiring and molecular-cellular activity, you continue to create more of the same. Yesterday's hardwired habits ensure that tomorrow will be a repeat of yesterday. If you want to heal yourself—become more whole and more integrated and improve your outer life of friends, family, career, and so on—then you have to begin to rewire yourself. You have to begin to evaluate and observe what is running through your head on a daily basis, as well as your emotional patterns and addictions.

If you're trying to lose weight, stop using alcohol, end an abusive relationship, or heal a physical pain or illness, you have to break the habits that are entrained into the nervous system. It's not easy, but it's very doable!

In general, these habits and patterns are entrained energetically—you are programmed like a computer. If you continue to always get the results you are seeking, keep on doing what you are doing. If you are not getting the results you desire in terms of health and relationships—personal or otherwise—you might want to change yourself from the inside out.

Emotional rushes—whether from stress, fear, anxiety, depression, or a fight or flight response—are naturally produced drugs with troubling side effects. These "stress and death" hormones are secreted in your body every time you get too upset about anything. Too upset means you are reactive, you are repressed or you feel stressed anxious, fearful, or otherwise not well.

Depression, repression, lethargy, low energy, physical pain, dissociation, and addiction to sex, drugs, or alcohol all point to internal struggles. Sleep problems, erectile dysfunction, excess anger, challenging menstrual cycles, etc., are indications of deeper subconscious patterns, emotional challenges, and addictions to stress and death hormones.

Instead of becoming overtly stressed, some people hold it all in until the pressure in the body gets to be too much. Then the body will act out in a million different possible combinations of disease. I have seen many people over the last thirty years in my private practice, and most come with some form of ache or pain or bodily dysfunction, but have no idea what they are feeling emotionally.

"How are you feeling?" I ask. "I feel pain," they say.

When I ask if they have any awareness of where in their body they are holding their breath or tension, few have any idea. When I begin to speak to the potential repressed emotions of the disease, they run around in circles mentally trying to deny to themselves that the physical disease has anything to do with emotion.

Think again!

When I ask, "What is your awareness of your thoughts? What do you find yourself thinking throughout the day?", some say, "I think about all kinds of things." Others say, "Not much." So I ask, "What thoughts are you aware of in terms of how you see yourself?" or "How do you feel about you?" Many will say, "I feel fine." Some will say, "Not so good, in fact I do not really like myself," which is more honest and a better starting point if it is true.

Healing cannot come from hiding. You must "know yourself," and if you don't, you would be wise to take the time to get to know yourself. This is important, because what you think and what you feel literally attracts the people, situations and circumstances that make up your life. You are a beacon of energy and you attract very specific people, places, things and events based on your overall energetic and emotional state. Remember, you are like a magnet. This, by the way, includes attracting bacteria and viruses. Certain energy dynamics, moods, etc., will cause various pathogens to grow out of control in the body.

When you realize that is how it is, it can be quite disturbing. It is mostly disturbing because it becomes quite clear that you have a lot of work to do. Many people come to the healing path hoping for physical healing, emotional salvation, freedom, and peace of mind. You can have all of that. Like most things of value, though, it rarely comes quickly or all at once—you have to work for it.

The hard part, at least initially, may be that it seems so daunting to unravel your complicated self and your complicated life. You are the source of that complication, not the world around you. That is hard wisdom. It is also great news, though, because if you can do something to change yourself that improves your physical health as well as the well-being of your outer world, you begin to realize your power.

## Changes in Health, Job, and Relationship

Obviously, some of us have more challenges than others, but most people are in deep need of healing even if they do not admit it and even if no one close to them notices. So many people are suffering and pretending they're not. People do what they think they have to do, what they think they are supposed to do; they follow all the rules. Then they can't figure out why their body is screaming at them, or why life seems to be forcing them out of their comfort zone and out of their job or a worn-out relationship. Others rebel against all the rules and try to defy the system, only to suffer a similar fate. So it can seem like these are the only choices.

Both of these positions are outward-focused, so neither is going to bring out your best, neither is going to bring deep contentment, and neither will lead you to inner acceptance, peace, and true fulfillment.

Do you feel disturbed by this discussion? If you do, it means that the disturbance is there and you have been keeping it hidden. This dialogue is intended to provoke some of that. How can you know yourself if all is hidden? If you are simply trying to play by society's rules and regulations then you will produce many internal and external grievances. Remember, "Seek not outside yourself."

How can you look inside and say, "That is an old worn-out thought that does not serve me anymore; I think I'll drop that one," if you do not even notice that you are carrying it around? The answer, of course, is that you can't.

How can you look at society and say "Wow, we are not really well; in fact, I think we are dysfunctional and I think society needs an overhaul," if you are burying your feelings and your personal truth?

## Change Yourself and What You Are Putting Out There

How can you drop a feeling of guilt, shame, or lack if you do not even realize that you are running it through you, feeling it, and growing that feeling? How can you make a significant change in the larger society if you do not change yourself first?

You are an amplifier—you amplify energy. It goes out to other people and interacts with their energy. If you know this, you can work to clean yourself up. Clean up what you are putting out there. How can you change and heal if you do not know yourself? Becoming familiar with what you are thinking, feeling, and putting out can be disturbing if you are sending out negative thoughts, moods, and energy.

It can also be awakening and empowering, though. What you can "catch" yourself doing, you can observe, rethink, reprogram in your body and send out as new, conscious, and improved messages. Every message sent is received by you in the moment you are sending it and by someone else too! So be conscious about what you are sending into the world.

Every person—whether they offer a positive or negative presence—is going to take others with them. Learn to think for yourself, heal yourself, better yourself, and you can make a difference in the world.

To heal yourself, you have to change your own hardwiring. You have to change your own energy and nervous system. You are like a walking magnet, and your thoughts, words, and feelings create an energetic, electromagnetic force that literally pulls certain people and circumstances into your life and repels others.

If you want to change your life for the better, you have to work with and on yourself! You have to take the time and energy to observe yourself and influence yourself as well as change what you mentally hold on to; what you think; and how you walk, talk, behave, and contribute to your world.

When you are conscious of what your thoughts mean to you, how you speak them aloud, and what they indicate about what you really believe, you can catch a glimpse of what you are putting out there and, therefore, what you are attracting in return.

In doing this—rather than just blaming others—you have the opportunity to send out new information, and that information will inevitably return with new feedback. Once you realize that your life, your personal reality today, is a reflection of what you believed life was yesterday, then if you do not like it in any way, you have no choice but to change you!

If you know that you thought it (consciously or haphazardly) and you subsequently attracted it into your world in the form of people, places, things, and events, and you were to own the fact that the law of attraction is always in effect, then you would know that it is you that must change first. Do not expect other people to change for you. Do not expect world peace from other people. You create it or it doesn't exist. If you are waiting for other people to change so that your life will get better, hunker down, because it could take a long, long time.

## Purifying the Body's Water

If all that makes sense to you—fantastic! Even if you're not quite sold, you might want to contemplate purifying your body's water and its associated energetic structure.

Your body is about 60% water. Your water has a molecular structure that can be seen under the microscope. It looks like beautiful crystal when it is healthy, but murky, dirty, and cracked when it is sick. See Dr. Masaru Emoto's book, *Hidden Messages in Water* to see what pictures of what water looks like at a molecular level when it is healthy and when it is sick.

In the meantime, consider what the research by Dr. Emoto and others demonstrates, which is that water is affected and programmed by consciousness, thoughts, words, prayers, and the like. Take a time out and look this information up on the Internet. See the images of how the structure of water at a molecular level is changed by simply writing the word love on your water bottle!

I am not here to convince you of the validity of this research, however. I am here to teach you to do a "hack" practice; to speak consciously and deliberately over your water! You have the power to change your water, down to the molecular level. This creates health and vitality or sickness depending on what you are up to.

Again your body is roughly 60%+ water. Your brain is more than 70% water, your blood is more than 90% water, and your cells are roughly 70% water. All of these are essential to your health and well-being. You are a walking vessel of charged water. What are you thinking, speaking, walking, and praying over your water—over your brain, your blood, your cells? Do you carry holy water around with you or dirty water?

You cannot curse over your water and expect it to be healthy. You cannot curse over your life and expect it to get better. When you curse over your water you are cursing over your life and vice versa.

Do you want greater health, greater energy, and greater power? Then purify your mind and your water! Do you have a water purifier at home? If not, it's worth the investment, given all the chemicals, pharmaceuticals, poisonous metals, etc. in many water supplies.

Just as importantly, what do you say over that water in your water bottle or your bathtub? And what about the water in your body? Your water is going with you wherever you go and it is influenced by you—the thinker, the speaker, and the consciousness! Like it or not, it is how it is. So you make the best of it or you make it worse. Choose wisely.

Do not panic—it's not good for your water! Instead of worrying, instead of reacting, begin wherever you are to consciously and deliberately program your water. I like to walk. Whether I am pacing my living room or walking out in nature, I like to literally speak over my water. Rather than letting my water just come along for an unconscious ride, I speak to my water consciously and deliberately as much as possible. I also speak over the water I put into my body. I also speak over the water in my bathtub. I speak to the water and consciously program the water that I offer to my plants, the water I place in my boiling pan, my coffee, my kombucha tea, my coconut water, etc.

## *Walking and Talking over Your Water Practice: Influencing Your Inner and Outer Reality*

Speak over your water, your body, your brain, your blood, your cells, and the water in them. Try this one: "I am strong, healthy and vibrant. I exude health, happiness, and longevity."

- Do not mumble! I cannot hear you! Shout it out! Walk it aloud like you yourself are going to part the Red Sea.
- In another moment, say it lovingly.
- Do not be attached to which one is working; both are speaking to your water. It will become what you tell it to, but not if you mumble to it.
- Ten minutes at least today!
- You program it if you try and you program it if you just mumble to yourself unconsciously.
- It does not matter that some part of you—what we might call ego or monkey mind—says, "This is stupid and it is not doing anything. I don't think anything has changed." So what? That is why I am telling you to look at Dr. Emoto's book and images on the Internet from his research just long enough to convince yourself this really happens! Because it does, even if you don't see result immediately.
- You are setting things in motion whether you're conscious of it or not, and, for the most part, it all takes time. So do not expect to see instant results from your practice. Initially, think in terms of thirty days. What kind of change can you produce in thirty days?

Say this: "I am strong, healthy, and vibrant. I exude health, happiness, and longevity." Now say this once or twice more to warm up, but do not stop there! If you understand that this is how it is—your thoughts program your water for health or disease every day—then you realize how important this practice is and you do it for longer and longer periods of your day, week, month, and year.

If you mumble and walk around with your head down as if you are not good enough and you are praying to someone or hoping for someone out there to agree with you, you are missing the boat!

- We are talking about water here. It listens and it adapts to how you are programming it. So walk for fifteen minutes. Walk for one hour and you have yourself a real power walk!
- If you are walking and swinging your arms and your head is down and you are thinking nonsense and you think that this alone is good for your heart, think again!
- Instead, hold your head up. Walk consciously, spine straight, with attitude! Do not ask your water, do not ask someone else's opinion, instead walk and speak out loud with authority: "I am strong, my body is strong, my mind is strong. My water is vibrant! I exude health and vitality!"

You can make up your own words and your own phrases or you can use these for yourself. Take ownership of them, though; do not mumble them and think that they will lead to magic. Talk directly to your water. Know that you are speaking things that are having a direct influence over the water in your brain, the water in your blood, the water in your cells and the water in your kidneys! If you carry a bottle of water with you then you are programming the water in your bottle as you walk and talk as well.

- "I feel utterly fantastic, my water is radiating vibrant health and my body feels healthy, energetic and refreshed."
- Take responsibility for what is running through your head, for what comes out of your mouth. Say it like you are commanding it and say it like you will not accept anything else!
- Belief is not required, except that you have seen enough of the science to keep trying.

When you practice qigong, when you practice meditation, when you play some soft soothing music, you are practicing and influencing your water. Stress, inflammation, fear, and pain are all signs of toxic water, toxic blood, and a toxic lymph system. Rather than chasing the symptoms around trying to get them to go away so you do not have to face yourself, clean up your stuff.

You cannot curse someone else without cursing yourself. It is true, physically. Curse someone else and you curse your own water. Bless someone else and you bless your own water.

Blessing your water or someone else's is not something that only priests can do. It can be done by anyone. This is being done in laboratories around the country; healers know it, shamans know it, and physicists know it. What if you were to subject yourself to positive thoughts, words, and sounds—do you think it would have an effect? You bet it would!

Check out Larry Dossey, M.D., and his book "The Power of Prayer," and check out all of the experiments that are mentioned and all of the results from those experiments. When you read some of those experiments you will once again have the evidence that human beings have greater power than they typically realize. That, though, is not enough, so I am saying to you to then come back to the practice. Look at the research; look at what it is suggesting and then come back to the practice! Without the practice, we just have research that tells us how great our potential is but if that is all we get out of it, so what? The objective is to make your life and the lives of others better. As Jesus said, "…whoever believes in me will do the works I have been doing, and they will do even greater things than these…" (John 14:12–14).

Do not worry about how often you are being "not so positive" or whatever that looks like to you. Conscious and deliberate power thinking, speaking, walking, and talking will always tip the scales and—in this case—your water, in your favor! Five minute and fifteen minute power walks and talking over your water several times over the course of a month is going to make a significant difference in your world. Subtle perhaps, but significant, especially if you keep it up.

## Recovery from Physical Injury or Sickness

If you have been knocked down by injury or physical illness, you may feel pretty distraught. If you cannot swim or run or lift weights or do your gymnastics or, for some people, even go for a walk, then you are physically down. You may also be "down" mentally and emotionally. This keeps the mind-body in a toxic state and makes it much harder for the body to heal itself.

Your mind programs your water! So instead of hoping that you will get better, instead of waiting eight weeks for your bones to heal, instead of fighting against your water, try speaking to it with some vim and vigor, with some attitude and enthusiasm and programming it consciously and deliberately. Walk and speak your way back to health and vitality. Use your mind even if you cannot use your body. If you have to drag one leg around while you walk and speak aloud in your living room telling your water how strong you are, then do it. Do it until your second leg agrees with the first one.

## A Personal Healing Story

I once broke my hand in three places during a martial arts demonstration. My hand was crumpled back to my wrist and I had broken three major bones. The surgeon wanted to place pins in my hand and told me that without them I would never be able to lift my three fingers again—they would all droop. I declined the pins, and he told me I would be back in eight weeks with a deformed hand. I came back in three-and-a-half weeks with healed bones and a healed hand. I now have full mobility and function, and the bones are stronger than they were before the accident! I spoke over that water, I spoke over that hand, and I told my body it was strong and I told my hand it was strong and I told my water that it was healthy and vital.

When I began that practice with my cast on, I didn't have a lot of confidence. I was, well, broken. Temporarily.

I picked myself up and I walked and I talked and I kept on moving on. And guess what? It passed on by. I left behind this terrible time to usher in a new and improved reality, a new and improved situation.

When I met that surgeon at the hospital, he was quite upset that I refused the pins in my hand. He was convinced he was doing me a disservice by letting me go without them. I could appreciate where he was coming from, but I had a plan and it worked.

When I returned and he took some x-rays, he was shocked! He said, "What do you do again?" I replied, "It is called qigong."

You can do it too! Talk to your life! Talk to your water! Bless it. Love it, heal it, make it great!

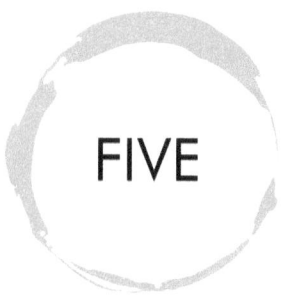

# FIVE

# THE ALCHEMIST

"The secret of life, though, is to fall seven times and to get up eight times." Paulo Coelho

Seeing yourself as an alchemist is a shift in attitude and perception. It is the shift from being a victim at the mercy of external circumstances—other people, bosses, jobs, financial worries, physical disease, etc.—to being the master of yourself, your body, and your personal reality. It is the shift from being anxious and worried to being fearless—you can learn to be fearless even in the face of fear.

Alchemists know they can turn any situation, any circumstance, and any problem into gold. I am primarily talking about metaphysical and metaphorical gold here, but these practices will also affect your ability to manifest physical and financial support, wealth, and abundance.

How you see things matters! How you see a situation matters! How you see yourself matters!

Alchemists know this and use it to their advantage. They contemplate these questions and answer them openly and honestly because if they can become conscious of the "heavy lead" in their energy field they can change their views, and, in so doing, turn that lead into gold.

## Journal Practice: Reframing Difficult Situations

Think of a situation you're struggling with.

- How do you see this situation? What does it mean to you?
- Write down the first answers that come to you.
- Once you've answered the questions, rewrite the answers and give the problem a new meaning.
- For example, if your original answer is, "This situation sucks—I feel so limited and taken advantage of," remind yourself that this is an attitude and a perception of victimhood and that it will continue to create conflict for you.
- If you practice qigong, you may be able to loosen your grip on this perception and attitude. You may be able to evolve the emotional attachments and addictions, and change the hardwiring that says this perception and this attitude are correct, justified, and real. You may also be able to direct energy toward a new thought, new attitude, and new perception. In this regard, I am referring to the physical practices of qigong as well as our power walking and talking exercises.
- Try rewriting your answer to something like this: "Although this situation appears to suck, I am learning the meaning of perseverance and patience. I know I do not belong here and I know this situation will pass—I am on the way to better things. I am grateful for what I have learned here even if the only thing I learned is that I don't like this."
- How do you see yourself right now? Be honest! How you truly feel about you is influencing your personal world of people, places, jobs, relationships, finances, etc. If you are struggling, it is more than likely you are harboring some not-so-nice thoughts about yourself. Write them down.

- For example, you might be thinking, "I'm upset with myself," "I'm an idiot," "I hate myself," "I am so stupid," "I am not good enough." You may uncover all of these thoughts and more. You may need to dig, because most people are not typically honest with themselves.

- For example, you might feel bad about an event that has arisen in your life. You tell yourself that you feel bad about yourself because of this event, but it's more likely the event has come into your life because you were already feeling bad. Then the event occurs, you feel even worse, and you use the event to beat up on yourself. The act of beating oneself up can be obvious such as "I am so stupid," or less obvious; you are just upset.

- Once you've identified these thoughts, though, you can begin to rewrite them.

- You can ask yourself "What am I learning from this?" "What is the lesson here?" If you realize the lesson is "I do not want this ever again," this is progress. Now, though, you need to walk and power talk about what your life is about to become! "I am going to be the next best-selling author! I am going to be successful, wealthy, and happy"—whatever it is for you. You can create your life's story, and—if you stick to your story—it will shift your world inside and out.

- It may not be as quick or as simple as shifting your perspective to "I love and appreciate myself for all that I am. I am a great gift to all." Over time, however, identifying thoughts that weigh heavily on you energetically—"I am not good enough," "I am unworthy," etc.—and changing them to something lighter can create new energetic and neural pathways.

Ding-ding-ding. I hope that rings the bell. You need to practice these things enough that they change the energy that courses through your nervous system. You have to impress these thoughts on your biology. Do not expect your biology or your ego to "get it" initially. It has no reference for what you are walking and talking any more than your computer could perform Microsoft Word functions without downloading the software.

It takes time and consistency to download these things, but you are worth it! Ever started a download on your computer but then the Internet goes down and your download does not go through? The software does not work unless the full program downloads, so you have to start the download again. If you keep working at it, one day you will get it downloaded. That is when your life changes for the better!

Take a break—work on your thoughts. When you are ready to get physical again, check out the next qigong exercise!

## Qigong Exercise: Change Your Mind

Stand in a horse stance. Bend your knees a bit to make it look like you are sitting on a horse. Let your arms float up from the waist and take a position like that of hugging a tree or holding a barrel. This is a power pose. It is a static position that you are going to hold for a minute or two (or three, or fifteen, or twenty). Every minute you hold it, you are saying "yes" to being strong, you are saying "yes" to having powerful posture, mentally, emotionally, and, of course, physically.

As you hold this pose and observe, you are going to experience physical changes. Just like you changed your mental posture in the above exercises by rewriting the script, you are now going to rewrite the script by changing your physical posture, which will affect your mental posture. Through those changes in posture, you are also speaking to the biochemistry of your body, to the emotional attitude of your nervous system.

Your body will begin to rebel against the pose by causing you discomfort. For every minute you stay in the pose past your comfort zone, you are transforming yourself in multiple dimensions—mentally, emotionally, and physically. If you continue to work at this transformation, you move into the spiritual dimension of the work. Be sure to relax as much as possible in spite of the tension you feel and experience. That is the secret. It takes practice so build up slowly. First two minutes, then five minutes, then ten, etc.

## Understanding Energy Dynamics

When you become a qigong practitioner, you become an alchemist. Some forms of qigong are more attuned to this teaching than others, but, in general, this is true. Working with your energy and understanding energy dynamics in relation to yourself and others is a true shortcut, one that allows you to evolve and gain valuable wisdom.

So many people are tired and say that they do not have enough time, energy, and/or money to study such things. This clearly demonstrates temporary ignorance, because the realization that we create our reality with our thoughts, words, breath (or lack of breath), etc., brings with it a sense of urgency to begin the process right now, right here.

You can focus on where you want to end up, but you have to be here now and alchemize what is here now to create the shift that will allow you to move forward and to move beyond the current obstacles whatever they may be.

Many people think struggling with the outer world helps this process, only to discover after a long and arduous journey that they did not accomplish what they were trying to accomplish. Hence the saying, "That which you resist persists." Others know struggle is not the answer, but they're not sure what to do so they become apathetic. Becoming apathetic is not going to help either, because it too is a form of resistance. It will only make matters worse.

As both psychologists and metaphysicians tell us, denial leads to projection. Whatever you project, you are trying to get rid of. The bad news is it does not go away. Instead, you attract more struggle, and it all appears to be outside of you when what you need is an inner shift.

As a qigong practitioner and alchemist, you would rather break these negative patterns and create new neural pathways for your thoughts to flow along. You look at the rubbish in your own head—the noise that is holding you back, holding you down, or making you feel depressed. You can question those thoughts, reprogram your mind, and give yourself a new perception, a new way of seeing the world. You do not have to be perfect at this; you do not have to believe one hundred percent in some new positive idea about yourself. You just have to begin.

Try choosing thoughts that glow like gold. Dump the thoughts that do not serve you and burn up the heavy emotional energy that accompanies those thoughts. As an alchemist, you do not have one technique or one mantra—you have hundreds. You learn that the path is not about arriving at some place or about having enough. It is about being prepared because of what lives in you. What lives in you are inner resources. What lives in you is the kingdom of heaven. There is no lack in the Infinite and the Infinite lives in you. Qigong, being an alchemist, is about turning inward and working with what is inside.

Imagine there is a great moment coming for you. It could be anything you might imagine as a great moment, but—if you are not ready for that moment, for that opportunity, if you do not have the skills to negotiate it—it will be lost to you. Being an alchemist means you are prepared and that no matter what comes your way, no matter what you are facing inside or (seemingly) outside yourself, you will have the skills to turn any situation into gold. If you are practiced, you turn negative thoughts into positive ones, you turn negative moods into positive ones, you turn heavy leaden moments into golden opportunities.

One of my spiritual elders once said to me, "There is no such thing as being ready ahead of time; instead, you show up to your life, you show up to your moment." Each time you do this you become better and better at turning inward and bringing forth what is needed in each and every one of your moments, each and every one of your challenges.

## Practicing Alchemy in the World

The need for skill, a strong practice, and the application of that practice to your life cannot be overestimated. Some people practice qigong once a week, twice a week, once a month, or once a day. You have to have some kind of core practice like this if you want to bring the practice into your daily life—into the bank, into your relationships, into your job. If you want to bring the calm of qigong to work, you have to practice qigong before and after work so that the calm becomes a part of you.

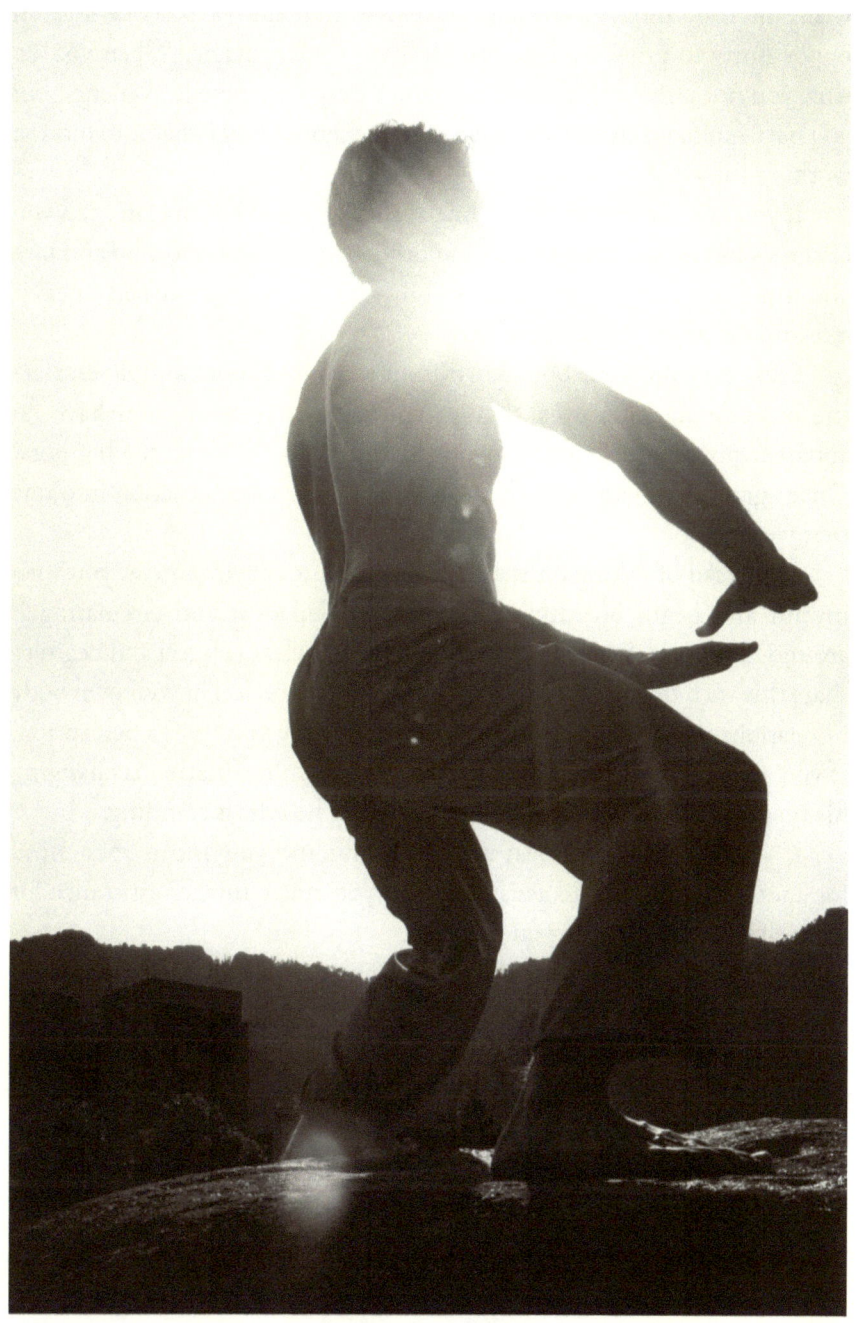

*Photo By: Lisa Siciliano*

Over time, as your mastery increases, you can make your entire day, week, month, and year—each and every moment—a practice and an opportunity to grow, evolve, heal, and work your magic. When you do this, you not only have a chance, you not only have potential energy, but you have momentum and you have kinetic energy, energy that is in motion working for you. You generate power!

If you are standing in a long line at the bank and you are late, can you create a shorter line, actually cause another bank teller to show up and save you time? You can, potentially, and—if you do—you just turned a heavy, stressful situation into a lighter one.

Can you calm your boss down from across the room and de-escalate the business meeting even though you are the secretary and have no apparent power to influence anyone in the room, let alone the big boss? Once again, if you are an alchemist, you can turn any situation into one that yields gold!

If, instead of taking on the stress of the outer environment, you turn inward and begin breathing imaginary golden dust and circulating it around the room; if you focus on how calm and clear you feel and begin to share this with the room, changing the heaviness you feel in your own body in relationship to the room, then you will change your boss's perception. If you are astute, then you will see that your own meditation is changing his breath, causing him to swallow, changing how he is standing.

If you are calm and clear and accepting and you ask in your mind for another bank teller to assist you, can you create further assistance for yourself? Potentially, yes, you can.

Might you still be late and somehow energetically change the rules of engagement so that when you show up to the meeting everyone will be okay with the fact that you are late? Yes, that is also possible. The key is to turn inward and work with what is within you.

Is it possible to shift the state of a client's illness to a state of healing? Of course it is.

If a client's energy is such that they are creating illness in their body, is it possible for me to change their energy system from one of heaviness to one that is as light as metaphorical gold? Yes, it is.

I must first connect to their energy system and have a common intention with them to bring healing. Once I do that, I can begin to speak quietly in my own mind to their energy system and say loving things, healing things. I can guide their emotional state into higher energetic states by holding particular mental postures that cause the energy to alchemize, evolve, and grow. There are many things we can do for ourselves and for others when we become true alchemists.

You may realize that your connection to yourself is primary and that all change and evolutionary growth begins there. You may also realize that your thoughts, words, deeds, perceptions, attitudes, and mental and bodily postures affect your energetic makeup. Your energetic makeup flows through your neural net and your entire nervous system, and that makes you a walking magnet. If you want to change anything, any situation in your world, breathe it in, change its heavy feelings within yourself to something lighter, and watch what happens around you. Watch what happens to the people around you.

You have the power to influence the world around you, and a good place to start is with yourself.

There is no better time than right here, right now. Do not try to escape your troubles or your problems—turn them into gold instead. That is your key to opening the door to a new reality. Love your neighbor, love your life, love your situation, even if you do not. Change your attitude toward it.

Break the habitual cycles of thought and what you feel when you think "I am not good enough," "I am not worthy," "They judge me," or even what you feel when you think you do not have enough money. Instead of sitting there in your stuff, break the cycle by thinking or doing something new. When "it" is happening and you are feeling it or you are hearing it in your head, do qigong, go running, tell yourself a new and improved story. Tell it how you want it to be. Don't fight or argue, shift it. Shift it inside yourself!

Do something different to break those old habits! Try the qigong habit instead.

## Qigong Practice: Power Walking and Talking

- So walk with me. Talk with me.
- Power walk it, power talk it.

Write the following on a piece of paper (or use your own words): "I am healthy, I am vibrant, my body exudes radiant health." Speak up! I cannot hear you!

Repeat: "I am healthy, I am vibrant, my body exudes radiant health." Speak up! I cannot hear you!

- Be loud, tell your body and mind what is up!
- Take the piece of paper for a walk right now (or as soon as you can) and read the script!
- Walk with your head up. Walk with your spine straight. Walk with a smile on your face and walk with attitude! Speak loudly. Then try speaking more softly but very, very clearly and deliberately.
- Reprogram, restructure that life of yours and watch what it does to your mood, watch what it does for your health, for your energy levels. If you make this practice a habit, you will reap so many benefits that currently seem unfathomable to you. Do not just take my word for it—walk it, talk it, own it!
- Let's do a ten-minute walk and let's have at it!
- And if you are brave and you are ready, let's do it once in the morning and once tonight and the same for tomorrow! Do this for the next few days and you have rocket fuel!

## Healing Benefits of This Exercise

If you're consistent and committed to it, this exercise can lead to a happier, healthier life. You can have cleaner, purified water running through your body, healthier tissues, better brain and memory function, greater immune function, cleaner blood, healthier organs, better cholesterol levels, and much more!

A lot of people will struggle with an exercise like this because they somehow believe they are unworthy of what they are asking for. They believe things like "I cannot have that" or "I don't deserve it." If that is you, when you finish this exercise you may still feel depressed. You might say to yourself "Well, I don't really feel much of any change." And if that is you, then you said it with your head down. You said it out of unworthiness.

A few notes on unworthiness:

- It is rubbish! We make it up!
- We can say we are unworthy and not do anything for our own benefit, but the whole time worthiness is in you—always has been, always will be. You always have a choice.
- The universe is unattached. It will give with or without limits. You can choose limits or you can choose to un-limit yourself.
- There is an old saying that you are created in the likeness of the Father. If your worthiness is ever questioned it is only by you, because science is proving that—whether you think you are worthy or not—you influence water! You influence plants. You influence bacteria. You influence light energy. You influence your life.
- So many of us feel that we do not deserve better things because someone else does not have them. Whether it is the starving children in Africa or your sister, many people feel guilty about the idea of improving themselves and their life circumstances. Another lie.
- If you better yourself or make yourself worse, either way you will take others with you! So please, for everyone's sake, better yourself!

If you had trouble with this exercise, walk it again! If you struggled with this exercise, I feel compassion for you—but I don't feel sorry for you—because you made a choice. I remember what it was like to be in constant pain. I remember what it was like to have fallen off the horse and to feel the pain, the unworthiness, etc. But I have no choice now but to urge you to pick your head up, stand up straight, and march on. This will work, but it takes time and consistent practice. It takes reprogramming.

What else do you have to do? You are always creating, and the world is always mirroring back to you your perception of things. So make good choices.

Remember, don't be disturbed when the universe does not fulfill your request simply because you asked three times. There is a reprogramming involved in this process. Be patient with yourself as you gain momentum!

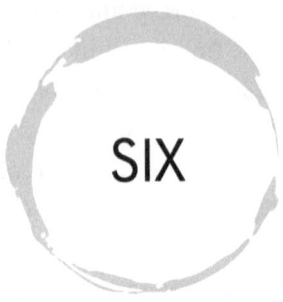

# SIX

# MASTER YOUR MOOD

"You are at a choice-point in every moment of each circumstance, each activity, spoken word, and thought."
Reverend Dr. Michael Beckwith

Your mood is another aspect of you, another level of you that you can either be owned by or that you can control. Control your mood—not through suppression or repression, but through conscious and deliberate programming—and you become a super-empowered human being!

Your mood is a great indicator of what your mind has been up to lately. Specifically, it's an indication of what you, the thinker, have been thinking.

Your mood is a biological state created by hormones and other cell-to-cell communicators. Initially, it comes on following a stream of consecutive thoughts (typically unconscious thoughts) that have built up momentum. That momentum is always headed in a particular direction.

We can never just observe an experiment or anything else and be impartial. We influence it! We also influence it in the direction that we intend to influence it! Your mood is not random. You are orchestrating it consciously or unconsciously, masterfully or not so masterfully.

Once momentum builds, follow-up thoughts will be produced in conjunction with the mood itself. If the thoughts started with so-called negative thinking, then they will create a bad mood and the follow-up thoughts have no choice but to become increasingly negative. Many people are not at all aware of what they are thinking until they are already in a bad mood and many more people will not realize it until their body becomes sick or they have an anxiety or panic attack or they are depressed or are in some other kind of unwanted emotional state. Repressed thoughts and emotions explode and override a person's ability to suppress them in panic attacks and they do the same with depression, except that the energy is turned more inward.

Some people do not notice what they are thinking and feeling until someone else does something to them that seems to disturb their "peace." They might then say, "I was doing fine until so-and-so did such-and-such and ruined my mood." The first thoughts are missed completely until the negative mood sets in. If this continues, you will attract other players in your outer world who will continue to "disturb your peace." They will seemingly interfere with you and your plans to be happy and live in peace and harmony.

If this happens to you frequently—or even occasionally—you might want to regain some control over yourself, your body, and your life. Negative thoughts drain your energy system. Negative thoughts lead to negative feelings and moods, and those moods will wreak havoc on every cell in your body. They will make the blood, the lymph system, and the water throughout the body and brain toxic. They will also affect your relationships, your work environment, and your bank account.

So say it with me, "Subconscious (and sometimes conscious) thoughts (and negative judgments) lead to moods, moods lead to secondary thoughts, and if I do not change what I am thinking, my mood and my thinking will progressively get worse."

Everybody has been in a bad mood. Ask yourself, "When I was in a bad mood last time, did anything positive occur to me during that bad mood?"

More often than not, bad moods lead to more troubling events, so getting out of a bad mood as soon as possible is of the utmost importance.

If you like bad things happening to you then by all means stay in a bad mood. The best way to attract "bad happenings" is to simply think very negatively about yourself and the world. This is of course a bad attitude that produces a negative mood that draws in the right players to help you play out that negativity.

The great news is that it works the other way too. Think positively enough, eliminate some inner demons and negative beliefs, adopt a positive attitude (as best you can), and you will begin to change your mood. Your mood is a beacon and an amazing magnet for attracting people, places, things, and events.

If you have positive thoughts leading to positive moods running your life, all is good! If not, you might want to get a handle on your subconscious and conscious thoughts as well as your mood. One place to begin this is by consciously and deliberately thinking over your water (see the Purifying the Body's Water section of CHAPTER FOUR: HEALING). Another way to do this is to begin a regular qigong exercise practice.

Until we become more aware, more conscious, more quiet, and more introspective, we will miss much of what we are thinking. It literally goes by without you consciously noticing. Your water, your blood, and your energy field, however, not only notice it, but are programmed by that unconscious thinking. So until you become more aware of what you are up to in the control tower of your thoughts and your brain—your awareness—you are going to have to work hard to turn your thoughts and your moods around.

This is especially hard for people who have themselves locked into a negative mood. When you are locked into a negative mood and you are unaware of having thought yourself into this mood in the first place, it can seem very difficult to turn things around.

The reason it seems so difficult is that when subconscious negative thoughts have created a mood, the mood then darkens the thoughts further. When the thoughts become heavier, so does the mood and you begin to attract situations, people, and circumstances that reflect your inner reality back to you. Ouch!

This can seem like a cruel universe at times. When you attract those challenges, the thinking mind says, "I can't believe he, she, or they did this to me. I can't believe they are doing this, that life is doing this." If the thinker, namely you, does not change your thoughts and your mood, you cannot escape the circumstances of your life. They just keep coming for you.

Do not fret! Clean things up. First of all, change your breathing, go outside, and practice some qigong exercises. Do a full twenty-minute or forty-minute routine. Then go for a power walk. Speak consciously, speak purposefully. Exercise your thinking to such a degree that it begins to change your biochemistry. When you think long enough, deliberately enough, whether you are being positive or negative, you are going to affect your biology. This is a fact. You are going to produce a mood. This mood is an attractive force and it will draw "mirrors" to you in the form of people who will play out different games with you. If your mood is negative, guess what kind of exchanges you will have with them?

Good actors and actresses can turn on and off certain moods. If you are an actor or actress, pay attention to the roles you are playing on stage, on television, or in the movies. Those roles will also affect your life outside your work, so be mindful of the roles you choose.

Even if you're not an actor or actress, if something unpleasant or unwelcome is happening in your life, pay attention. Rather than simply seeking a solution somewhere outside of yourself, take responsibility for the role you are playing in your personal movie. Notice what you are attracting, and if you do not like it, consider mastering an improved mood. When you are locked into problems and challenges and your mood is negative, it can seem like your mood is negative because of external circumstances. If circumstances changed, your mood would be great, or so you think.

Here's the problem: if you do not change your mood, the circumstances may not go away, shift, evolve, or change. So you have to change your thinking and you have to change that mood. The hardest time to do this is when you are "down." Taking on qigong practice, power walking and talking, and other new roles is easy when you already feel great. When you do not feel great and life has got you down for whatever reason, it becomes significantly more challenging to do these practices. Oprah Winfrey and Tony Robbins do not need these practices; for the most part they already have a great momentum going for them. So both of them, for example, actively practice an attitude of gratitude. It keeps them focused on the good in their lives and keeps them going in the direction that they desire to go.

If you are struggling because your success is not there quite yet, or you just are not feeling the gratitude thing, or even if the attitude of gratitude is one of your practices, qigong practice and walking and talking over your body can help you get centered, focused, self-empowered, and headed in the right direction. This effort will also help you attract even more to be grateful for into your life.

A lot of spiritual teachers and gurus like to focus on the gratitude piece, and I agree that it is an important aspect of the journey. I also know, however, that, again, the hardest times to do these practices are when you feel down. Perhaps your parents, teachers, and experiences as a kid taught you that you are less than you are, and, as a result, you think that and feel that and build relationships around that.

Then you end up angry and create a life that, on multiple levels, offers significantly less than you feel you deserve. Maybe your relationships are subpar, maybe your job is subpar, maybe your finances are subpar.

Then along comes the teaching of gratitude and it just makes you angrier. Maybe you hear Oprah talking about how grateful she is and you think how easy it would be to be grateful if you were Oprah, but your life is a mess.

During challenging times, gratitude is a great practice but that doesn't mean it's easy. You can create a better life for yourself and march yourself out of what you've settled for. That is what I did, so that is how I teach you to do it.

## *Qigong Exercise: Walking*

- Walk consciously and stay focused and connected to the earth with each step. Bring your awareness down to your center of gravity, your lower dantian.
- Walk and talk out loud: "My life is great. My life is headed in a fantastic direction. Great things are happening for me." Say it like you mean it!
- One time is nothing. Say it twenty-five times (or 100) then take a deep breath!
- If you feel like crap, speaking these words is hard; it is like pulling teeth for some people. But if you understand how the chain

of events unfolds, you have no choice; you must change your thinking by choosing new thoughts right now. Speaking them aloud makes them even more effective.

- You have to do the practice until it changes how you feel—that is the secret! Think it, speak it, and walk it until it changes your mood. How long does that take? One minute, one day, or one week, do it until you feel the shift in your mood, because until you shift your mood you have not shifted your energy. Until you shift your energy, you cannot positively influence your outer reality effectively.

- Get a piece of paper or copy, paste and print: "My life is great. My life is headed in a fantastic direction. Great things are happening for me!" Repeat, repeat, repeat. Repeat it 100, 1,000 times.

  o Read the "script" until you feel it! Until you believe it, at least a little, but the more the better.

  o As silly as this may sound, you are on stage and you are in a play. If you do not like the role you are playing, change it. Rewrite your script. Once you rewrite your script, you must act it out. Practice in such a way that it is your job to get the director to hire you. If you are now taking on the role of a positive, happy, successful, and healthy person, then you have to become that. You have to act that well enough that the director wants to hire you for the part. When the imaginary director says, "That is the best presentation of a positive, happy, and successful person I have ever seen," you have created what you were looking for.

  o As much as this is an act, you will attract more of whatever you hold in your mind—happiness, for example—because you are by nature an amplifier.

- Another way you can do this practice is to pretend that you are on the phone. In fact, pick up your phone and put it to your ear.

  o Pretend your friend has called you and they have asked you how you are doing. Respond by saying: "My life is great. My life is headed in a fantastic direction. Great things are happening for me!"

o Then pretend a second person calls. Tell the first person you have to go. Tell them thanks for calling and take the next call. Pretend the person on the phone asks you how you are doing. Respond to them in the same way: "My life is great. My life is headed in a fantastic direction. Great things are happening for me! Thank you for calling I have to take this next call.

o Again, you say, "Oh yes, I am doing great! Thanks for calling. Yes, my life is great. My life is headed in a fantastic direction. Great things are happening for me!"

- If you look into the research on this you will see that the brain does not know whether you are pretending or whether this is a real event that is happening to you. Either way your body will begin to respond as if positive events are happening for you, even if they have not really happened for you yet!

### Qigong Practice: Laughing

Laughing is amazing for your liver! Your liver detoxifies your blood. You need it. It needs you. Laughter can be something that you can do now; do not wait for some funny business, be funny for the health of it right now! Laughter can also draw more auspicious people, places, things, and events into your life, so why wait?

Some important research on smiling and laughter has shown that four-year-old children smile and laugh about 400 times a day, while adults smile and laugh only 14 times a day. Wow!

In general, kids are much happier and less stressed out than adults. Can you purposefully laugh for the health benefit of it? Can you smile for the health benefit of it and get the same effects in your biochemistry? Of course you can.

You have heard the saying, "fake it until you make it!" Through the power of laughter, people have healed cancer, reduced heart disease, and diminished stress and anxiety.

Why wait until a moment comes to make you happy? Instead, just choose to laugh it up for the health of it! Qigong is the skilled cultivation of universal life force. Laughter qigong involves influencing that life force through the skilled practice of laughter. It takes time to become a good laughter practitioner. Many studies have shown that laughter produces a surplus of endorphins, which can decrease your pain and elevate your mood.

So, what are you waiting for? Bust out in laughter, show those pearly whites. Does anyone know a good joke?

- Hold your hands over the right side of your upper belly by your ribs. Your liver is located near that area. As you hold your hands there you will practice laughing aloud: "Ha Ha Ha Ha Ha."
- Start with one minute, which can be challenging for some people. Have you ever laughed so hard it hurt? That is so good for your liver; fake it until you crack yourself up.

Laughter can also lighten up your attitude and mood. If you are upset about some person or some event or you are struggling to resolve an issue, you'll likely have a very difficult time laughing about it. If you have a serious health issue that may keep you from a weekend sports event, and you've been training for more than a year, do you think you could laugh about it? Not unless you understand this type of practice.

Laughter is medicine. Laughter changes your mood. If you change your mood, you change your inner world. If you change your inner world, you change your outer reality. This gives you an option you may not have known you have.

When you decide you have a problem that cannot be resolved easily, you perpetuate that problem. Learning to laugh despite your problems and being silly like Jim Carrey would be is a form of alchemy that can change your mood. One of my students had an issue with his hip. It was a serious issue to him and was inhibiting his golf game. He learned to laugh about it, have fun with it and not take it so seriously. This, along with some other qigong practices, allowed him to win the club championship more than once.

So, for now, just try it. Go back and read this exercise aloud and try it out. Even if your life does not radically change because of it, you will change what is flowing in your blood after just a few minutes of practice. That is great medicine!

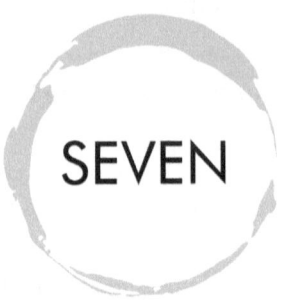

# SEVEN

# PRIMARY THINKING VERSUS SECONDARY THINKING

"I now command my subconscious mind to direct me to helping as many people as possible today to better their lives by giving me the strength, the emotion, the persuasion, the humor, the brevity, whatever it takes to show these people and get these people to change their lives now." Tony Robbins

Most people are not conscious creators, but rather are living their lives in such a way that they react to what they are experiencing. If you are one of those people, you fight against those experiences and the people you think are assaulting you, and base your future decisions on those upsetting events.

You wake up in the morning and let your body tell you whether you are happy or tired or sick or well or whether you have a lot of energy or a little. Reactionary thought is secondary thought. It is based on some feedback that you are getting from your body or from your external personal life. Maybe someone insinuates that you are looking older and then you begin thinking that maybe you are. Your body feels tired or feels old, and you get out of bed and your mind says, "I am getting old." This is secondary thinking.

Maybe your job has not been going well and it begins to fall apart, your lover wants to break up with you, your car is breaking down and you think "What the hell did I do wrong?" This too is an example of secondary or reactionary thinking.

It takes time and work to realize that you may be thinking things; you may be having unconscious conversations with people. You may be lining up events. If you are saying things about yourself in a not-so-positive way and you are creating heavy moods, then you are going to see that reflected back to you by your outer world. You then experience these bodily and emotional reactions and you further exacerbate them by fighting against them and thinking things like "Where the hell did that come from?" as if you are being attacked by an outside force.

You may then make the mistake of blaming the mirror. You are then perhaps angry with the person or the event that is bothering you. You react by fighting against this person or this event that appears to be outside of you, attacking you.

Some teachings say that you must give up control—"Give it up to God" Or "Give it up to the Holy Spirit." When you cannot think straight and people or places or things are coming at you, this is actually a wise idea, a practice of least resistance, of surrender.

There are things you can control, however. There are things that you can master and—if you do—you can control them. If you control them, you align your mind in such a way that existence gives you back more of what you are aligning with. If that is happiness, then you get more of that. If it is being centered in nonresistance—which you might think of as meditation or the practice of observing without getting lost in the reaction—then you will tend to dissolve situations because you do not make them any worse by resisting them. You must do this internally—not simply intellectually, but energetically and emotionally.

Life is a mirror, whether you like it or not. It will mirror back to you what you have been thinking, musing, meditating on, fretting over, or getting excited about. Or a mixed bag of all of it, if that is what you are putting out there.

This is hard wisdom, and it may take some years to get your mind around it. If you no longer wish to experience certain things, then you can no longer afford to think them, run the old programs, live the old habits, and expect things to change. Until you can slow things down enough to get a handle on what you are doing and what you are creating—in the moment you are creating it—you need to begin to interrupt these negative vicious cycles as a conscious practice.

This needs to be done preventatively when possible and when something arises in your outer world that seems to attack your inner peace, remember that you can always make it worse. Or you can begin dissolving it by dealing with yourself, your thoughts, your energy, your reactions, and their associated emotions.

Creating dysfunctional karma, blaming something outside yourself and then reliving it over and over again like the movie *Groundhog Day* is not good for your health. The body cannot handle it—it will begin to fall apart at the seams.

So you have to interrupt this trick you play on yourself. Instead of disowning what you have created, whether it is a bad hair day or a low energy day or a money-less day, you need to own it and simultaneously interrupt its momentum. You need to deal with your emotional reactions and your reactionary thinking.

If you resist it, fight against it, and blame it, you perpetuate it. Instead, let's talk about primary thinking and how you can use primary thinking to get more of what you want and less of what you do not want.

To use primary thinking, you have to be a little cocky, as Bruce Lee liked to say. He liked the word cocky. I do, too. Primary thinking, unlike secondary thinking, has nothing to do with the current state of any situation. Secondary thinking is always based on the current state of a situation and your reaction to that state. Primary thinking can be thought of as unconditional, unlimited thinking. It can also be thought of as thinking that is done over bodily situations, emotional states, circumstances, problems, challenges, and the like. On the other hand, secondary thinking says, "Oh crud, this is how it is and this is how it will be forever and I am screwed and once this settles in things will be really,

really bad, because then what will happen next is that I will have to do this, this, and this."

Primary thinking can dare to look at that and laugh and say "Not in my world. Ha Ha Ha, I feel great, I feel grateful, and I love all of the really great people I meet each and every day!" You should know by now that saying this one time after a troubling event has upset you is not going to stop your negative momentum in its tracks and shift you to a positive frame of mind. Yet, when is a good time to begin getting on the right track? The best time is ahead of time, right? Until you become like Tony Robbins or another positive idol, you will be creating trouble for yourself along the way and you will have to work to get over that trouble, through that trouble. If you're smart, you will want to do that as quickly and as efficiently as possible. You will want to get on the right track as soon as you possibly can.

In the beginning, your challenge will be the perception that life and people and places and things are attacking you. You had a say in it before it happened but maybe you missed that part. Now you have this challenge in front of you and—let's face it—your attitude about it is not great.

That is what you must work hard to correct. You could have used primary thinking initially, and maybe you did use it by putting some positive vibes out into the world. Maybe, though, you were not aware of some of your inner demons and your negative beliefs, and now they have shown up in some dude named Bob. Now you have to deal with Bob.

Secondary thinking will be reactionary, it will fight against Bob and whatever problem you have with him. You could keep playing all that out and make it worse and worse for both you and Bob. Or you can begin rewriting the script right now.

"I love the people coming into my life. Around every new corner comes a new best friend. I love people. Have I ever told you all how much I love people? I love them. They are so beautiful and wonderful and helpful!"

You can tell the story like that even in the presence of a challenging story and a challenging person. In such cases, even if you had already created conflict with a guy named Bob, watch what happens. If you are sincere and successful, you will change that relationship on the spot. He will see you differently and you will see him differently. What was a bad situation will give rise to a better one. It all starts with how you perceive it, label it, and live it.

## *Primary Thinking Practice: Breathe and Rewrite*

- When you see a negative cycle occurring, first take three deep breaths.
- Take three deep breaths right now before continuing or you will not do it later.
- Pause.
- Once you have taken three deep breaths to slow it all down, use your primary thinking.
- Think over the situation. Write a new script over it.
- Try this: "I am an infinite mind, living in infinite possibility. There are infinite solutions to this little obstacle. In fact, I am so much bigger than this little obstacle that I need do nothing to fix it. I say it fixes itself."
- Say this twenty-five times. Each time say it louder with more enthusiasm.
- Later, every time you think about it, which is secondary thinking or reactionary thinking, you say "I expect it to fix itself. I expect it to fix itself. It has fixed itself."
- Again, "I am an infinite mind, living in infinite possibility. There are infinite solutions to this little challenge I am experiencing."

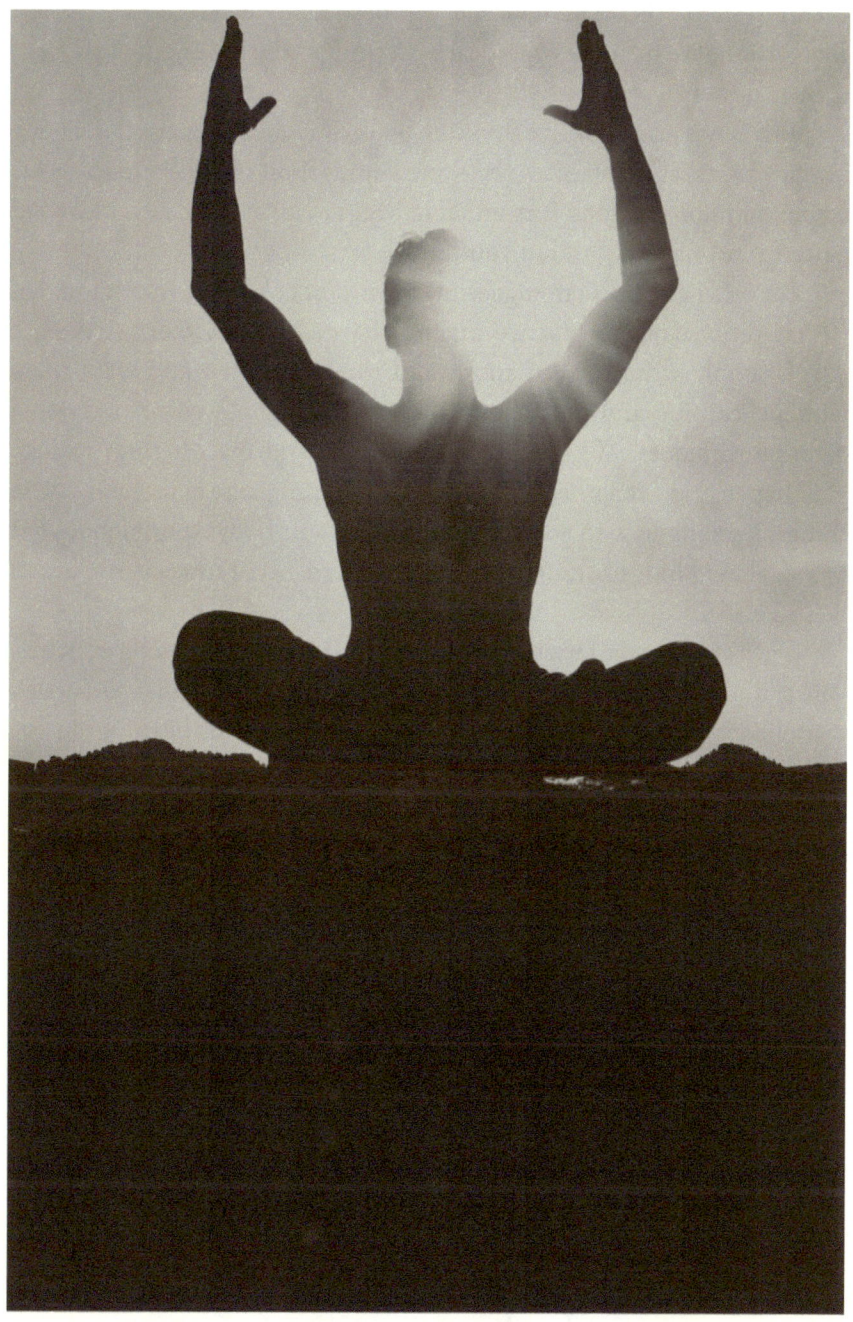

*Photo By: Lisa Siciliano*

Remember, everything you do either adds to or takes away from your energy system. The more depleted you become by overreacting, the less energy you have to create or to deal with things. The less energy you have, the less powerful you are.

This is not just a positive thinking book. It is about qigong and qigong is a practice that emphasizes the skilled cultivation of chi. Practicing the actual traditional qigong is essential to begin to anchor the new ideas and patterns in your body and in your breath.

The other exercises I'm suggesting are meant to be done in conjunction with traditional qigong practice. You may have a less satisfactory experience if you simply write these mantras and thoughts down and walk them without learning and practicing energy gathering and other traditional qigong techniques. We developed our online and live offerings to help you deepen and strengthen your practice. Breathing and embodying these things, learning how to control your breath, your body, your blood, your mood, these kinds of things must be practiced 1,000 times if you are to be successful.

Once you are comfortable with and skilled at the core qigong exercises, you can also integrate these other hack practices (shortcuts) to further consolidate your gains. Otherwise, you run the risk of burning up the energy you gathered to yourself during your qigong practices. Qigong exercises are great by themselves, but coupled with mind and mood control, for example, they can help you create a better life for yourself on many levels and in many arenas.

When you are creating your life, thinking ahead and trying to be positive, do your best. Simultaneously, when life seems to throw you curve balls and you cannot figure out where they came from or what you were thinking that might have created them, use primary thinking to change the circumstances of that situation on the spot.

If and when you cannot even think straight, get back to physical qigong exercises, take three breaths, and clear your mind so that you can get yourself back on track. Then return to using this type of thinking again as you feel more empowered to do so.

If you have a health condition and you wake up in the morning, drag yourself out of bed, and say, "There it is again, God damn it!" you are perpetuating that condition. So make a different choice and practice qigong right then and there. Then maybe go for a power walk and tell life what you expect to see occurring in your world next.

As they say in *Star Wars*, "I am one with the Force. The Force is with me." Think about it—it doesn't say the Force is against you; it says the Force is with you.

Jesus said, "My mind and my Father's mind are one." He didn't say that life was against him.

The old program, the ego, the monkey mind, your past, your past relationships that played out in conflict—all of that may have been against you, but that is not your higher path. That is not your destiny. Your destiny is greater than that. My destiny is greater than that. Evolution does not simply repeat and repeat all the while you are being pummeled by something outside of you. This may be how it appears sometimes, but that interpretation can only come from temporary confusion.

### Primary Thinking Practice: When You Wake Up in the Morning

- "Today is a new day. Today is going to be different because I say so. I am my body's master; my body is not my master. I am strong, my body is strong, because my mind is strong. I feel great. I feel amazing. I feel freakin' fantastic!

  Oh my God, today is brilliant! So awesome that I am going to meet new people today. So awesome that people love me just the way I am. So awesome that I am so healthy and that I have so much energy! Oh my God, I feel good!"
- If you can be a little silly with this, you will lighten your mood and be successful.
- This will not work if you are determined to be a sourpuss. It's your choice.
- I dare you to be daring and say it for the fun of it, because you can!
- Try saying this for seven days in a row, first thing when you wake up in the morning.
- Make note of what happens.

One of the biggest challenges you may face with current situations in your life is that you believe that they are not transmutable. This can keep you stuck in situations that are long overdue for a change. If you feel it, see it, smell it, then you are in it and you may not be able to see beyond it. But your mind can be the ship that leads you to different waters.

It is not simply about the words or prayers that you say. They have no power if they have no meaning to you. They fall on deaf ears if you have no passion for them. It is not about changing God's mind about you or the universe's mind about you, it is about changing your mind about you and your situation or circumstances.

As many spiritual teachers remind us, the universe always says yes. It always agrees. Remember, though, that it doesn't respond to your words as much as it responds to your feelings. And what drives your feelings? Your thoughts.

Be cocky. Dare to speak things over your life, over your flesh, over your biology, and do it even when you would typically curse yourself, curse your body. That is the rubbish that has to stop!

Every time you make a mistake or try something new and curse yourself for trying, you have to catch that habit and you have to do something new and different. The words fall flat unless they change how you think and feel about yourself. They fall flat unless they change how you feel about yourself in relationship to whatever it is that you are speaking to, whether it is your health or a relationship or your career.

Many of us have never been taught to love ourselves. Such a simple thing, but think about it for a minute. Did anyone ever teach you to do it? You learned math, you learned English or Spanish, but did you learn to love yourself? Self-love is absolutely part of the equation here and is essential for healing and our collective evolution.

Let's face it, this is a workout. In many ways it's like going to the gym. Training your body is important, but your mind is your greatest asset. The rest is either interference or adds to the equation. Your body, its biology, your mood, your emotions, your secondary thoughts are all secondary. Your mind, though, is primary and is the essential ingredient. Lazy mind is always reacting and living from reaction. Learning to find creative and influential mind—primary mind—is key to making a difference for the better in your life.

Don't forget that life is magical. Don't be dumbed down by advertising that bombards you with all that you supposedly lack. Lack of health, lack of fitness, lack of money, lack of makeup, lack of beauty. Just get outside and breathe again, reconnect to nature.

Stop. Slow down. Come back to yourself. Take back your power.

Go look into your son's or daughter's eyes, take three minutes. Just look at the stars instead of watching television tonight. You have to face what you are connected to and what you are putting out there. What you are sending out into the world—you will see it reflected back every day.

You may have all kinds of excuses for sending out trouble, anger, frustration, depression, etc., etc., etc., but what if you accept that what you send out comes back to you. Truly. If the law of karma is true, the law of cause and effect is real and operating, then, like Bill Murray's character in *Groundhog Day,* you have no choice but to change what you are sending out into the world.

The temptation is to get caught up in projection, blame, confusion, amnesia, sleep, unconsciousness, etc., and ignorance is bliss until it is not. Ignorance is a common approach for many people: "If I ignore these problems, they will go away."

That which you resist, persists; it doesn't work to ignore things. You can move from here to there, you can hide and avoid, but wherever you go, there you are. That is the universe's justice. The universe wants everything to evolve. Look around, read some books on biology or physics. The universe wants you to grow and evolve, not ignore, burn out, and fade away.

When you become like Bill Murray's character in *Groundhog Day,* you realize you cannot get ahead through any false attempts, manipulation, coercion, or even self-destruction. They do not work. There you are and there you remain and there your life is until you change from within.

One day, many years ago, a negative event happened to me. I felt abused, taken advantage of, mistreated, and victimized. But I had been journal writing and trying to become conscious of what I was creating in my world. When I took my three deep breaths and reminded myself that I was an infinite mind living in infinite possibility and that my thoughts, feelings, and energy were attracting my experiences, I remembered something. I remembered something I said, who I said it to, and when I said it, and I knew that this experience was a direct reflection of what I had thought. I also felt it and spoke it out loud to a friend in the car the night prior to this event. I knew beyond a doubt I had attracted this event.

My volatile reactionary feelings and secondary thoughts did not last long. I was actually overjoyed to realize that I was creating my personal reality! I immediately thanked the universe for the experience and said "No more!" I would rather know myself differently.

After that, I started having more positive meetings and exchanges. In my experience, the universe will bring you positive exchanges just as readily as it will bring you negative experiences. We have a say and we have a choice which it will be. As Jesus said "As we sow, so shall we reap."

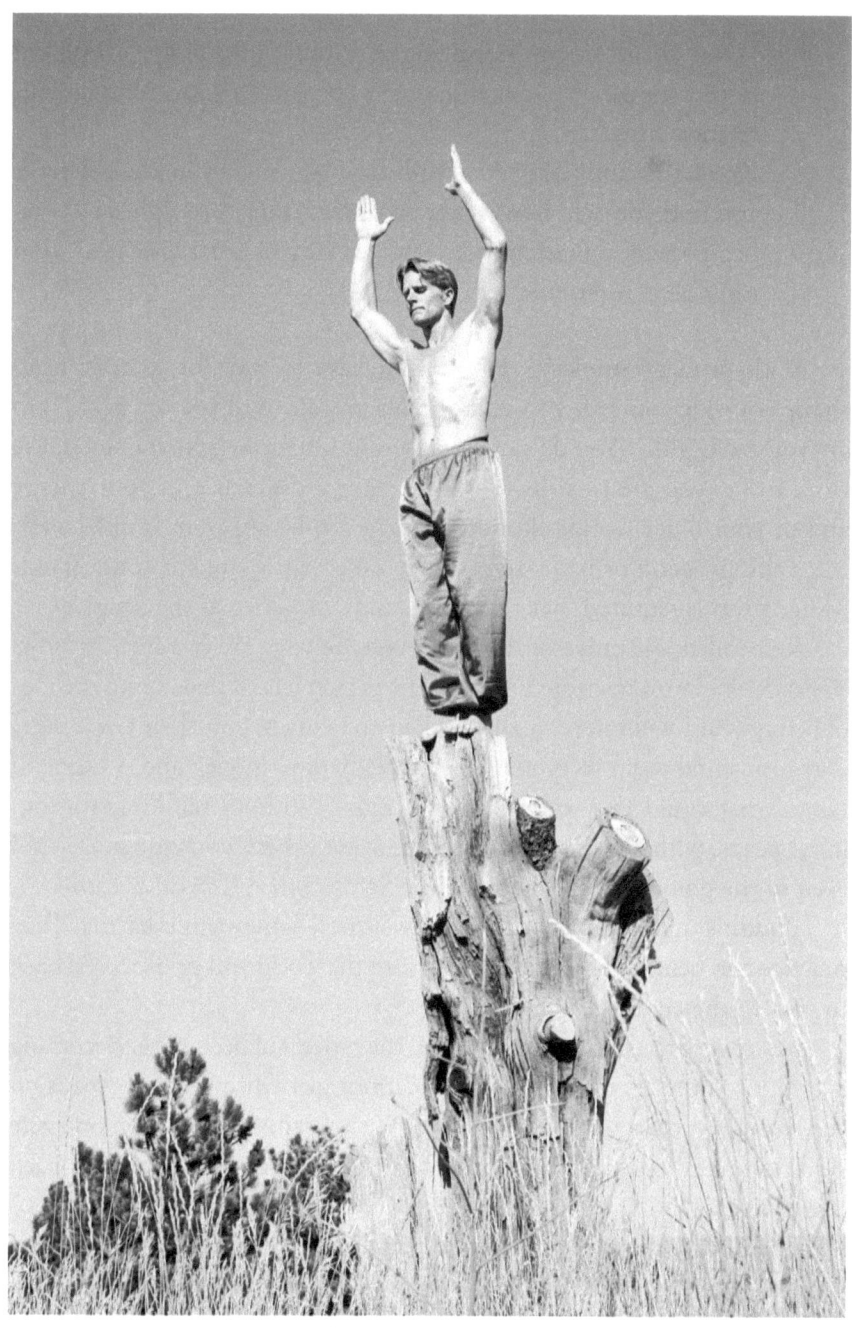

*Photo By: Lisa Siciliano*

Try this again:

- "I am an infinite mind, living in infinite possibility. I love and respect myself. I am grateful for kind people, friends, and conscious relationships."
- Know this and then act accordingly. Wherever you are, wherever you find yourself, however good or bad things are right now, you begin to set in motion what you are going to experience next from right here, right now.

With primary thinking, you do not have to wait for something to change outside yourself. You do not have to wait until you are healthy to say you are healthy. You do not have to wait until you have money in the bank to say you are wealthy. You can make a difference in your energy and in your outer world, although it may not be apparent immediately. Most things, good or bad, aren't—they take a little time to come about. Momentum is required, whether it serves the negative or the positive.

Remember, the universe always says yes. So what are you creating now? What do you want to create next? For the person who is dialed into the idea of being wealthy but never really worked on being happy, their *Groundhog Day* is pushing them to evolve. They already have money and power and fame, what could they possibly want, right? Without self-love, without inner peace, without love and appreciation for others, you will feel fearful even to the point of being haunted like Scrooge in *A Christmas Carol*.

Buddhist monks work with this law as well—they call it karma. They practice and believe that what you put into the world will be mirrored back to you, so they practice consciously.

Many wise teachers say we are all in the process of becoming. Becoming is evolution, the art of evolving. You cannot just whisper a few words on the wind and then whisper or shout ten thousand more in the opposite direction and honestly blame the universe because it is giving you back mixed signs.

The Buddhist monk or nun who prays for serenity must offer serenity, must think in terms of serenity over his or her own body, his or her own water. They must think serenity over the negative emotions that arise because someone did something that caused an internal upset, a reaction.

They can use primary thinking to think over it and shift the energy of it. They pray and chant for peace and calm their own minds, and this in turn calms their bodies. They are practicing changing themselves to also change the world. Some of these entities take on a great responsibility for the condition of the world and they are on a mission to change it from the inside out.

## Beyond Physical Qigong Exercises

There are many physical qigong exercises for physical health and mental and emotional well-being. Most of them are more easily conveyed through live or video instruction.

Qigong traditionally means the skilled cultivation of universal life force or chi. A more expansive understanding, though, leads to the awareness that you are organizing the energy around you with your thoughts, words, actions, and deeds. Physical practice is only one aspect of qigong, and there are many other exercises and healing rituals that can accompany the physical practice. The following practices fit in that category.

Remember that all of your actions and deeds are either gathering energy to you or depleting it. Depleted energy means fatigue, lack of longevity and ill health. So if you seek to better yourself, you must be more conscious about your own actions toward yourself, others and your environment. Through conscious and deliberate lifestyle choices and actions, you can make a difference in your own life as well as the lives of those around you.

### *Primary Thinking Practice: Giving and Receiving*

Try this exercise for offering goodness and receiving its effects. This can be done over any negative thinking you might be experiencing. It can be done over your depression and anxiety, and, if you do it enough, you will shift your lower vibrational energetic state from the heaviness alchemists associate with lead into the lighter, more refined energetic states associated with gold.

I recommend you copy and paste this on a piece of paper and take it for a walk.

"I offer you love, light, joy, kindness, compassion, exponential healing and eternal peace."

- Pick a person in your life and speak this to them on the level of the mind—the human Internet—or speak it aloud in your private space or outside. Speak it directly to them on the level of the mind only.
- Do this for at least ten minutes.
- After ten minutes or longer how do you feel?
- How do you feel?
- If you do this with sincerity you will inevitably feel lighter.
- This is a selfless practice that will also heal you.
- Try doing this over the course of thirty days with someone you can observe and communicate with during that time. You will more than likely see and hear about improvements in their life and/or situation. If not, do it for another thirty days.
- I offer long distance healing around the world on a regular basis. This is one of the types of practices that I do for each person signed up for the monthly healing programs. It has powerful effects because we are all connected.

Read this next section and know that I am speaking this to you. Please sit down and take three deep breaths. This is for you:

> To you, my beloved reader, I offer you love, I offer you light, I offer you joy, I offer you kindness, I offer you compassion, I offer you exponential healing. I offer you eternal peace.

> Again, I offer you love, I offer you light, I offer you joy, I offer you kindness, I offer you compassion, I offer you exponential healing. I offer you eternal peace.

> Again, I offer you love, I offer you light, I offer you joy, I offer you kindness, I offer you compassion, I offer you exponential healing. I offer you eternal peace.

Again, I offer you love, I offer you light, I offer you joy, I offer you kindness, I offer you compassion, I offer you exponential healing. I offer you eternal peace.

Again, I offer you love, I offer you light, I offer you joy, I offer you kindness, I offer you compassion, I offer you exponential healing. I offer you eternal peace.

Again, I offer you love, I offer you light, I offer you joy, I offer you kindness, I offer you compassion, I offer you exponential healing. I offer you eternal peace.

Again, I offer you love, I offer you light, I offer you joy, I offer you kindness, I offer you compassion, I offer you exponential healing. I offer you eternal peace.

Again, I offer you love, I offer you light, I offer you joy, I offer you kindness, I offer you compassion, I offer you exponential healing. I offer you eternal peace.

And again, I offer you love, I offer you light, I offer you joy, I offer you kindness, I offer you compassion, I offer you exponential healing. I offer you eternal peace.

And yet again, I offer you love, I offer you light, I offer you joy, I offer you kindness, I offer you compassion, I offer you exponential healing. I offer you eternal peace.

Now take a deep breath. Pause a moment. Ask yourself: How do I feel?

In this exercise, primary thinking is used to think over the thoughts, feelings, and energy dynamics of what is occurring in your consciousness and in your body. Whatever you think that reality is, that solid reality, it is transmutable. You can transmute your reality by using primary thought and not getting lost in secondary thinking, reactions, and secondary energetic states that have arisen because of those old thinking patterns.

Physical qigong exercises can be very helpful in breaking these cycles when you simply cannot think clearly anymore. Breathing, exhaling, moving the body, and consciously stilling the body can break these secondary thoughts up, because it changes the energy dynamics and the way energy runs through the nervous system. These secondary thoughts have loops or neural nets—they are ingrained patterns and can be very difficult to disrupt.

They can be interrupted, though, and it is worth the effort. Simultaneously, realize that this work is great work. It does not just happen because you mumble a few things and then you arrive and now you can go back to doing what you were doing. This is transformational healing; it is about the evolution of your consciousness, of energy, and of who you think you are. This takes work—it is an endeavor. That is why I have taken the time to write a whole book about it and why there are so many different practices here for you to try.

Famous rappers, for example, who focus their thoughts, feelings and beliefs on money, cars, and girls can and do attract that. They can literally go from broke to rich, sometimes very rich.

Many other business-minded people have created empires. When it comes to health and longevity, however, many of these same people will have meteoric rises followed by hard falls.

True healing and transformation for you, your neighbors, your friends, and your family—as well as the health and well-being of the planet— requires a deeper and subtler understanding of the healing process. As you evolve, you have to take others with you. Self-love and love of others has to be part of the equation.

Otherwise, you will inevitably step on others on your way to success. They will resent it, you will feel guilty, and it will come back to bite you in the end. So living consciously is your best offense.

As a personality, an ego, a separation-minded person, you can change your image, your clothes, the words you speak, the thoughts you think. You can take on a new character, play new roles, and change the surface of your life. You can go from broke to rich, from obscure to famous. But if healing and wholeness is not part of the equation, if self-love and love of others is not part of the equation, your success may be short-lived.

Healing is about win-win. Healing is about deep contentment that does not and cannot come from some thing, some place, or some state outside of us. This is what teachers mean, in my opinion, when they say, "seek not outside yourself." To seek, to be, and to have, I think, is most appropriate. But if you are wise, you do this for everyone in a practice of inclusion and exponential giving. The focus is on win-win; unity consciousness; the healing of others through disciplines like massage therapy, acupuncture, and medical qigong; and teaching others qigong exercise and how to better their lives.

These practices and others like them can bring contentment, inner purpose, friends, and soul mates that you would otherwise not attract. Even if you are not involved in the healing arts, sharing your spiritual and material abundance enriches your life and the lives of those around you. As you learn to love your neighbor you will also learn to love yourself.

As your practice and understanding deepens, you will find yourself thinking thoughts like "I am an infinite mind, living in infinite possibility and in infinite energy, and I am alive and aware and grateful."

If you are thinking that, more often than not you are going to meet some awesome people! You are going to have some awesome relationships! You are not just going to get some stuff or have a nice house that you have to hire security to protect. You are not just going to sit in your nice home and feel lonely because you are so rich and so great and no one likes you. You will not have to sit in your $5 million home and get drunk just so you can feel okay about yourself.

Exercising some degree of unconditional love is something else entirely. It is about cocreation; it is about the power of two minds being greater than one because they have joined together to expand and evolve life itself. Primary thinking can lead you and the others around you to such a reality. In fact, it is your destiny to uplift your neighborhood. World peace is a fantastic idea, but it begins with people like you and me setting higher standards for living and being—first and foremost for ourselves.

Remember the Tony Robbins quote at the beginning of this chapter: "I now command my subconscious mind to direct me to helping as many people as possible today to better their lives by giving me the strength, the emotion, the persuasion, the humor, the brevity, whatever it takes to show these people and get these people to change their lives now."

Whether you like Tony Robbins' style or not, you might have to admit he has done some amazing things for many people. He is very successful in many people's eyes and also very rich. Look at his quote, though, and how much he emphasizes being helpful to other people. This type of declaration is one that places an emphasis on win-win and exponential growth for the benefit of all, including Robbins himself. To me, this is beautiful. I am more of a healer than a salesperson or a businessman, but regardless of what role you choose to play in your life, you might want to include other people's success along with your own in that equation.

### Primary Thinking Practice: Thinking Over Your Secondary Thinking

Primary thinking is what you have the power to do at any moment you choose. Secondary thinking is past-based reactionary thinking that is limited in its perception. Secondary thinking knows nothing of infinite possibility, but it thinks it knows everything. It uses its limited perception of the past to dictate and determine the future. You can see how this could be problematic.

Secondary thinking says, "I do not feel like getting out of bed today." Primary thinking has the power to agree or to say, "I dare say, I feel awesome today!"

Secondary thinking says, "The cup is half full." Primary thinking can agree or say, "I see the cup as overflowing!"

Secondary thinking based on your past experiences wins out when you decide that no other options exist for you. You—the thinker—then recreate your past by thinking the same old stuff that you thought to create your past in the first place. If you think it again and feel it again and wallow in it again you will attract it again and again and again. You are doing this to yourself and there is no evolution in sight, only a loop called yesterday.

To me, the Beatles song *Yesterday* is one of the most depressing songs ever written, but it does describe what the past can feel like. If you would rather feel differently, you need to think differently and you need to do that right over how you feel. Change that thought process and, with enough effort, you will change how you feel.

The song *I Feel Good,* by James Brown has a very different vibe to it. It has a different train of thought driving the song, and the instruments that complement the song create a very different effect. If you want to see for yourself, listen to the song *Yesterday* by the Beatles and then listen to James Brown sing *I Feel Good*. You will most likely understand what I am getting at.

Both of those songs could be used to start your day, and each would create and attract very different experiences for you. Don't believe me; try it for yourself. Listen to one of those songs several times in one day and then ask yourself how you feel. Also make a note of what happened that day and be sure to take note of what happens the following day after those thoughts and vibes have caught up with you.

## Becoming the Supreme Grandmaster Creator of Your Personal Reality

The next time you are feeling down, limited, confused, or like life is pushing you around, throw some cold water on your face, get outside, and confront yourself, your inner demons, your old thought patterns. Wake yourself up to the greater reality of things.

Here are a few suggestions for you; you can use mine or create your own. Write it down or copy, paste, and print it, then take it on a power walk:

"I am the supreme grandmaster creator of my personal reality and I have total dominion over my life. I take total responsibility for the fact that I am where I am, how I am. I have done this to myself. In this moment I change my mind!"

"I choose radiant health, I choose wealth and prosperity!"

"I can choose to be broke and broken and I can choose to exalt myself. In this moment I exalt myself and all that I am and I rise to the occasion called my life!"

"I cannot be stopped from creating all that I desire to create and I create it in the name of all sentient beings, that all beings may experience their greatness without limitations, so be it!"

## Discovering Purpose in Your Life

Now, you might say these mantras or something like them but not follow through. Having a purpose in your life, a reason to get up every day, is extremely important! Forget about what you were taught growing up for a moment. You were created in the likeness of the creator, which means you have the ability to create. A rock does not. You do. Your divine purpose is to create. If you do not like what you have or what you are creating, create it anew.

This is why I love teaching qigong. It allows me to have a purpose and a career and get my own practice in on a daily basis, which I know is so important! It takes time to sit down and create or recreate your life. It takes effort and energy to think through how you might do it differently, but that is your divine purpose!

If you are doing a job you hate or going to college for a degree that you are not sure will accomplish what the college or your parents think it will, then think again. Create something new. I love to teach qigong because it allows me to focus on my own healing and self-improvement while taking many others with me. Also being a medical qigong healing practitioner and life coach with a private practice creates an ongoing flow of new clients who can benefit from my services.

When I teach workshops around the country, I'm offering others the opportunity to live the lifestyle that I enjoy. As my students go back to their neighborhoods and spread the healing, it benefits many more people than I could reach on my own—a win-win for everyone.

So many careers—including Western medicine, which I studied for a time—require that students sacrifice their health and well-being to provide healing to others. The more I realized that, the more I looked for a better way. I found it in teaching qigong and providing deep healing through medical qigong treatments.

To sum up:

- The secret with primary thinking is to be cocky and do it with authority. It takes time, but do not mumble and do not beg. Do not be angry and do not be sad. When you can say it without heaviness, worry, fear, guilt, shame, sadness, and grief, you will give to life a clear primary thought without conflict and the manifestation that comes back to you will reflect that.
- Go out into your life and follow through. Go seek and go find. Go with attitude and purpose and passion, and if you do not have

any yet, practice a qigong exercise routine until you do. Then come back and speak with some enthusiasm!

- Remember you are talking to your body and the energy. It's not better or bigger than who you are.
- Think about this—you are not talking to a God outside of you or even to the universe. You are talking to your biology and telling it to change, to vibrate differently. The great law, the law of karma, the law of physics, is going to take care of the rest. This takes practice, but have fun with it. You do not have to become a master overnight, nor will you. Keep working it. Keep practicing. Being alive is a great opportunity!

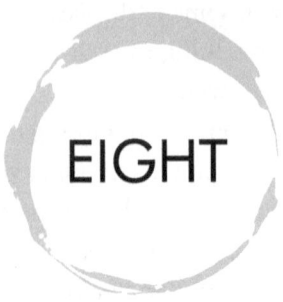

# EIGHT

# CHANGE YOUR BODY'S STORY

"We are what we think. All that we are arises with our thoughts. With our thoughts, we make our world."
Buddha

Your body is a feedback mechanism, just like your mood. It is an indicator of what is going on within you the thinker, you the feeler, and you the physical being. When you are unaware of your thoughts, your feelings, your moods, and your energy, you will often succumb to sickness and disease. If you do not listen to the disease and act on it accordingly, then you may end up with a serious illness, which is much more difficult to heal. Your body's aches and pains, colds and flus, injuries, and so on all have a story they are telling. In fact, the story they tell echoes what the body was told yesterday. If you are working on healing yourself, you might want to look into what the current story is and then change it. Reprogram it.

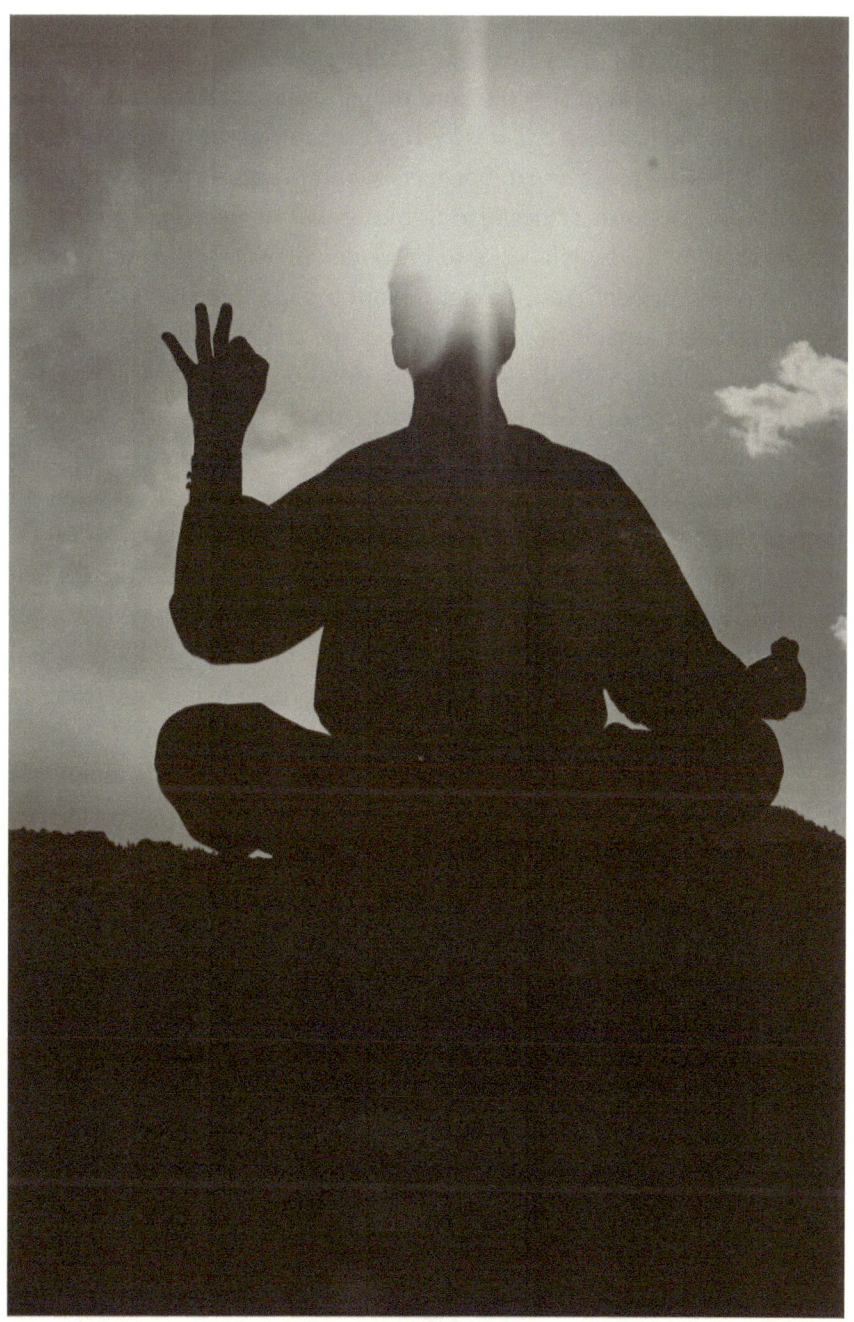

*Photo By: Lisa Siciliano*

If your body has some type of discomfort, ache, pain, or troubling condition, it is speaking to you. The worse the condition, the louder it is speaking to you. The story the body is telling is really an echo of sorts. It is the echo of what your subconscious thoughts have been, it is an echo of what your mood has been and it is feeding back to you the information you have been storing in its blood, bone, cells, and tissues. If the information has come in the form of negative thinking, heavy emotions, and dense energy, then the body will begin to break down. Where the body breaks down is never random. Your thoughts, your moods, and your energy play themselves out in specific ways and in very specific places in your body.

If you are not well physically, your mind is not well. The mind is always the source of what is going on in the body. If you develop an ailment from a chemical spill at work—and if you are sincere—you must take responsibility for why you were there in that moment to come in contact with that chemical. Even if someone else spilled the chemical on you, why did they decide on an unconscious level to be right there when the chemical spilled and not on the other side of the building where they usually hang out at noon on Tuesdays? This takes a lot of raw honesty and a lot of advanced healing work and introspection, but it's something to think about.

When someone falls off a bicycle, do they land on a random area of their body or is it specific? When someone becomes ill, why do they get breast cancer and not something else? Physical disease may not be as random as you think. I have worked with many people and their bodies, and I have listened quietly to the stories that were being told from the energy that ran in, around, and through their knee, their stomach, their back, or their hip. I found that all of these body parts and, more importantly, the consciousness associated with these body parts, were telling a story. If consciousness can program a body part with a story in the first place, then consciousness can change the story being told to that body part and eventually change the condition itself.

Here are some examples of stories that I have heard from people's bodies over the years. If your particular condition happens to be on the list, I am sure this will speak to you directly. Even if your condition or challenge is not on this list, what is most important to me is that you understand the concept, because then you can apply it to the practice of healing yourself, no matter what kind of challenge you are facing. Each story may be a bit different and yet each story has common ingredients.

## Physical Conditions and the Stories They Tell

- *Anxiety:* "I am worried about my future because of my past." "My past is coming for me and I cannot escape it." Even deeper might be the whisper: "I am guilty, it is all my fault."
- *Back Pain:* Is often associated with burden. I have heard many phrases in the energy makeup: "I am burdened." "It is all on me." "This is such a heavy load I carry." And different parts of the back can tell slightly different stories.
- *Upper Back and Neck:* "I have to control this." "I am losing control." I have also heard the opposite with the same effect on the upper shoulders, neck and back, which is "I am in control."
- *Lower Back:* "I am not supported." "Life does not support me." "My family does not support me." "I have no financial security." "I feel so unsupported." "I just can't do it by myself." And more.
- *Bladder:* "I am so pissed off."
- *Broken Limb:* "Something had to give." "I am fed up." "I feel trapped." "I have limited options." "I am limited." "I am broken." "I need to slow down." "Too much pressure!"
- *Cold:* "I am losing it." "I cannot keep it together." "I am freaking out." "Everybody just stay away from me." "I need to just get out of here but I cannot afford to." "I need a vacation but do not have the time." "I need to rest but I cannot afford to." "I just cannot take it anymore." "I am so stressed."
- *Cancer:* "It's all their fault." "I don't feel anything." I can't feel, I am numb." "I loathe myself." "I will never feel again." "I cannot nourish myself." "I do not deserve to be nourished." "I hate my sexuality." "I hate my prostate and my sexual desires, they were wrong." "Stupid uterus. I hate you, I hate myself for being a woman." "I cannot even stand being in my skin." "I hate my body."
- *Eye Problems:* "I am afraid to see what is right in front of me." "I am afraid to see my future." "I am tired." "I don't really want to

know." "I am sick and tired of this." "I am just going to tune out and fade away." "Who cares."

- *Foot Problem:* "I just cannot stand this." "I cannot move forward it hurts too much." "Trepidation consumes me." "I am fearful to move forward." Every step I take is painful." "I am getting old, so there is no sense in trying." "I cannot move."

- *Flu:* "I am just disgusted." "I am enraged." "I hate myself." "I feel so guilty for all of this." "Screw this." "I need to just cocoon and burn it up." "Everybody just stay away from me." "This is all my fault."

- *Headache:* "I feel like I am going to burst." "I cannot handle the pressure." "I am going to pop." "I cannot contain it anymore." "I am silent in my rage."

- *Heart Issues:* "I cannot feel love." "I have lost my joy." "I am dead." "I am heavy." "I am numb." "I am deeply stressed." "I am heavy in mind and in heart, it is hard to exist." "I am without passion." "I have no purpose." "I have no joy."

- *Hemorrhoids:* "I am enraged." "Life is such a strain." "Life is a pain in my ass." "She is a pain in my ass." "I need to get this done." "I do not have enough time to myself."

- *Hip Problems:* "I cannot negotiate this." "I cannot take my life in stride." "Too much fluidity is dangerous." "I have to hold back my fear." "I repress this sexuality." "I need to protect my pelvis." "I am not walking on stable ground." "Moving across the earth is a burden." "I am terrified." "I am enraged." (Note that terror and rage go together here and people can swing from one to the other.)

- *Impotence:* "I am nothing." "I am empty." "I cannot feel anything." "I am afraid to feel anything." "I am a shame." "I am afraid to be humiliated again."

- *Knee Problems:* "I am not stable." "I cannot trust myself." "I cannot stand in my power." "I don't like unpredictability." "My mother doesn't support me." "My father doesn't support me." "I feel unsafe about changing directions."

- *Lung Issues:* "I hurt so much." "My grief is unbearable." "Underneath it all I know it is all my fault." "I am guilty." "There must be something wrong with me." "I do not deserve to breathe." "I am disconnected from my spirit." "I cannot accept this environment." "I am at odds with my environment." "I am heavy." "I am hopeless."

- *Muscle Rip or Tear:* "I am vulnerable." "I am weak." "I am vulnerable to attack." "I am falling apart." "I cannot take it anymore."
- *Open Wound:* "I have been cut by life." "Life is dangerous." "I could die." "I am vulnerable, I am weak." "Get this negative ooze out of me."
- *Right Elbow:* "This is not funny." "Why is life moving so fast." "I cannot keep up." "Damn it." "I hate this stupid body." "Changing directions is not easy for me."
- *Shoulder Injury:* "I cannot shoulder it, push it anymore." "I cannot carry it." "I cannot handle the load." "I am not that flexible." "I cannot open my heart to that, it is too dangerous." "See I knew I should not have trusted this."
- *Tooth Abscess:* "I am worried that I cannot face this." "I am worried that I will not be able to get through it." "I am afraid I have bitten off more than I can chew."

Notice that each condition has a whisper or several whispers associated with it. In some cases, there are obvious correlations that can be made such as back pain and burden. In other cases, you might have to dig a little deeper to discover the grief in the lungs and even deeper still to discover the guilt that may be underneath that.

Each body part or condition has its story line. It is important to realize that the story line began some time ago. Do not expect to rewrite these stories by mumbling a few positive phrases once in a while. These are beliefs. Beliefs must be worked with in order to change to them, and this takes time and effort. It is important to realize that these conditions, these body challenges, did not arise overnight and may not go away overnight. The good news and bad news—but mostly good news—is that the body, as well as its cells, tissues, water, organs, and bones, is programmable. Its energy is programmable. Its DNA and its gene expression are programmable.

If you have a health issue that is manifesting in your foot, then knowing what is being whispered to your foot by your own subconscious mind is important. It is important to know what you are whispering to your foot so you can change that message, reprogram it, and heal that foot.

Not only that, but the foot or the back or the liver all represent something to your mind. The foot does what? It holds you up, it helps you walk, it helps you to move forward in your life. It helps you to stand tall. If it is not working properly it will not only affect how you stand—it will affect your relationships, your next move, your new job, etc. Every body part is related to your life in some way.

You do not have to figure out exactly what your foot is saying, but think about it. Think about it if your stomach hurts all the time. What does the stomach do? It digests food. What about your life experiences? How is it digesting those? Not so well. Then you need to do something about that so that you can find greater flow in the entirety of your life.

Again, most people are not aware of what they are thinking. They are also not aware of what they are feeling, emoting, and aligning with energetically. In time, when you know yourself better, you will see your deepest thoughts more clearly. Then you can ask yourself whether or not you want to entertain that thought, because you will know that every thought has consequences. You will also know that all thoughts you harbor are a choice. If you hold the thought subconsciously and do not ever catch a glimpse of what you are carrying around, then there is no way to change it. Once you see it, you can begin to work with it.

So many people have built their lives so that they never have time for introspection. What if that is what your life is supposed to be all about? What if life is mirroring things back to you so that you can see what you are thinking and feeling and subsequently manifesting so that you have the chance every day to do it anew? I would suggest to you that is a big part of what life is really about, so if you do not take the opportunity to do that and evolve yourself, you are missing out on life.

Your personal life is not going to get better because you finally got your degree, or got married, or are making more money. It is about knowing yourself and knowing what you are thinking about you that is then mirroring you back to you every day. If you do not like it, don't fight against it; just change it from the inside out. Easier said than done, but doable and well worth the effort.

## *Body Story Practice: Consciously Change That Story!*

Ask yourself, or your knee, or your back: "What do you think about this? What is this pain trying to tell me?" Journal write for an hour, asking questions and writing down answers.

Most of you will hear phrases right away that say things like, "slow down," or "take a break," or "lighten up," or "I hate my body," or "I hate myself." Whatever you hear, make a note of it. So if you realize your knee is saying slow down and rest, but you decide you cannot afford to, then you hurt yourself more. Even though you "could not afford to," you are now forced to and it would have been easier if you had listened to yourself sooner.

So make a note of what is being said and reprogram it. Offer the knee, the tissues, the cells, etc., a new set of messages. Also, make a note that you would be wise to make time for yourself! You'll have to if you want to make progress in your practices—it all takes time.

When in doubt, practice qigong. Breathe, move, practice stillness. Until you create the time and have the desire or the courage to do this type of work, practice the qigong exercises.

Repeat after me: "I am an infinite mind, living in infinite energy and infinite possibility, and I say that my knee (hip, back, eye, etc.) is healed! There is no problem here. There is no story!"

Then go practice qigong! Qigong by itself at your local YMCA is not enough. Just walking and making declarations is not enough but if you put them together you will get stronger and stronger!

This is easier said and done once than it is to repeat it until you see your condition, your situation, or your circumstance change. Remember— if, for example, it is your foot—your foot is connected to your job, your relationships, and your next move. So if you are going to change all of it in one shot, which you have the power to do, you need momentum of thought, new feelings, a new mood, and new energy patterns. Does that begin with one power walk and talk? You bet it does. Couple the power walk and talk with your qigong practice and you create momentum.

Do this mindfulness exercise one hundred times. You can do it in one, two, or four sessions. You decide. But know this—you need quality and quantity.

"I am an infinite mind, living in infinite energy and infinite possibility and I say that my knee (hip, back, eye, etc.) is healed! There is no problem here. There is no story!"

If you were to halfheartedly pray this to the sky, you would not get very far. Instead, say it over your biology. Say it over your life. Let your foot hear it, let the universe hear it, let your boss and your lover hear it across the ethers. Most importantly, rewrite the story being told over your biology.

Then do a ten-minute tree meditation during which you simply stand like a tree in the forest with arms down at your sides and be very still for ten minutes. To your monkey mind, this is a waste of time, but it is a very chi generating and healing exercise!

## Keep Changing That Story

Go for a walk, and while you are walking, standing straight and tall and dragging that foot—or whatever other problem you happen to have—along with you, say:

"I have always been strong, my mind is strong, my foot is strong, the bones in my foot are strong. Every single step I take is becoming easier and easier. I stand on solid ground. My life is improving exponentially every single day!"

Do your best to say this with some enthusiasm as if it is real. Remember, become a good actor or actress, play the role that you wish you were playing, and it might just become a reality for you.

- Get out a piece of paper and write this down or copy, paste, and print.
- Now take this on a walk and repeat it over and over and over again—100 times—so you can see the power of thought and how thought can and will change a mood.
- If this did not change your mood, do not fret! Walk it again until you shift it! Don't be afraid of a mood. It is an energetic, emotional state and you have the power to shift it!
- If it takes three minutes, two days, or two weeks, do it!
- Don't be concerned about the physical issue too much, it came from a bad mood, so more of a bad mood is not going to help.

Change the thoughts, change the story, change the mood. If you change the mood, you will change your state of health, you will change your work environment, you will manifest more of what you want because you focused on it and rewrote the story.

In these exercises and in your understanding, you now realize every condition; every health challenge has a story, and you now realize this story has to change. You have to realize that the body and its water and its cells and tissues are influenced by you, your thoughts, your moods, your energy dynamics. If you have been talking negatively over your foot for ten years, you have some work to do. I know because—as I mentioned in the introduction to this book—I had a severe spinal disease that the doctors said would cripple me. I seemingly got it overnight because of an "accident," and then I had to spend years getting rid of it. It seemed impossible, and I had to continually convince myself that I was an infinite mind, not a limited one. I had to convince myself that infinite possibility was the greater reality and that I wanted to and could tap into it. I had to stop praying to something over there, up there, or down there and realize that it's all here now.

Great teachings and spiritual truths and metaphysical science do not belong on some shelf somewhere—they are to be embodied. When you walk these thoughts over your foot, over your water, you are also walking them over your life. Your greatest obstacle is not your particular challenge it is that you believe in it. You believe in it more than you did before you had it. You believe in it more than you believe in any other reality. So you are going to have to convince yourself and your biology that a different reality exists and you are going to have to purposefully think thoughts and walk your walk, all the while facing your own disbelief that says the only reality is the limitation. It may be true that the limitation is now present in your life, but nothing is solid. It is all transmutable. It took time to create, it will take time to undo.

Many people say to me, "You don't know what it is like to have this and this." Actually, I do. I know what it is like to be told you cannot heal something, to be told that something is impossible. I know what it is like to have proof that says, "I am broke, I am broken."

But everything is capable of change, especially you. Instead of fearing change, change. Change for the better. Change to be healthier. Change to be wise. Walk it, breathe it, qigong it, into your body. Make your body healthy. Talk to it differently, walk in it differently, breathe it differently.

Maybe you do not think you deserve health. Maybe you and everybody else would just be better off if you were ill. Think again! It is a choice. Perhaps healthy, happy, and vibrant seems to be the harder choice from your perspective, but believe me, it is not harder. It is easier than being broke and broken, hurt or hurting.

## Bonus Practice: Healing a Sports or Other Injury

Do you want to heal a sports injury? Maybe you have fallen and broken something? Maybe you have a broken limb or an injury from cutting yourself at work and it will not heal? Or maybe you are a teacher or coach and you want to help a client heal. (If you are a teacher and/or coach and you want to help another person to heal, teach them the following). Here are a few healing tips:

- First, immediately stop talking about the issue (the injury, the illness, etc.).
- Only tell other people on a need-to-know basis. If they are not the doctor and they already know you injured yourself and they ask you how it is, tell them it is great and change the subject right away.
- Telling stories over your body is already happening. When you tell them out loud to someone else you are speaking over your body, over your energy, over your life.
- Be careful what you say and how you say it and to whom.
- If you want sympathy you want to remain sick. You do! If you want to be well then you point your mind in a different direction. A direction of health and wellness is not supported by telling people about your troubling health condition, so stop doing that right away.
- If people you've already told ask about your foot, A great way to respond is "What foot?" You can then say, "Oh yes, that…it is completely healed!"

- Your mind may think, "I am lying." You can think of it that way
if you wish, but you can also think of it as creating what you want
in the only moment that exists, which is right now. Say it and tell
it how you want it to be!

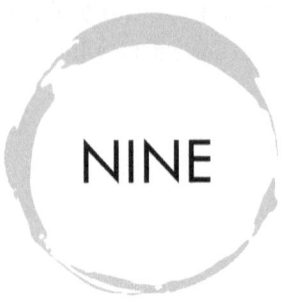

# NINE

# THE FORCE

> "For my ally is the Force, and a powerful ally it is."
> Yoda, Star Wars

Qigong is traditionally defined as the skilled cultivation of universal life force. It is a practice of harnessing universal life force or chi. This life force is referred to in the movie *Star Wars* as The Force. Yoda lifts a space ship out of the mud and throws bad guys without touching them. This is fun to watch at the movies, but has little to do with most people's everyday realities. Qigong can bridge that gap. Maybe you will not be lifting any spaceships anytime soon with touch or no touch but you may use The Force to heal yourself or facilitate healing for your family, friends and clients like I have.

Qigong is a form of exercise that can be done in the park and it is a practice that can heal your body. It is also a practice that develops your strength on a multitude of levels. Please see our Qigong Videos on Amazon: Titles Include Qigong for Beginners, Qigong Challenge, Qigong for Energy, Qigong for Stress Reduction, Chi Fitness and Qigong for Weight Loss. Be sure to search by title and by my last name Coon.

Once you have practiced qigong for yourself and harnessed your energy—harnessed the force of nature and of existence—you do not want to diminish your energy reserves by thinking, speaking, and acting unconsciously and/or negatively. Aside from other problems these habits might cause you, they deplete your life force, rob you of vital energy, and negatively affect your health.

I understand that this can be a daunting task on any average day, depending on your current life challenges. Having said that, show up! Do it! Master your thoughts! Master your moods! Do your best.

Everything you do either adds to or takes away from your energy system. Practicing qigong exercise is an important part of the equation, but so is living consciously.

Many people come to qigong later in life. Most of us are not eighteen anymore (if you are, welcome to the practice!). Regardless of your age, you might be interested in qigong practices that can make you feel like you are eighteen again.

When the average person turns eighteen, they begin to age more rapidly. The thymus gland, which is part of the endocrine (hormone) system, begins to shrink, and its functions are diminished. Remember that hormones are cell-to-cell communicators; they deliver messages of regeneration and life or messages of aging and death. Your thoughts and words impact your body all the way down to the cellular level. Most of us think unconsciously and therefore habitually, so becoming the master of your life and becoming aware of habitual thinking is absolutely essential.

When you practice qigong, you are exercising something that is more powerful than secondary thought, namely attention and intention. I touched on this in the context of speaking over your water and/or your blood and over your life in general, but what is its relevance to practicing qigong?

Remember the body is hardwired for chi. It is a conduit for electrical charge and the body's health and well-being depend on the smooth flow of this force in, around, and through the body. When you practice qigong exercise movements, you do so first with attention and intention. From there you move the body with a mindfulness that allows you to synchronize your mind, your body, and your breath.

The combination of exercising attention, intention, watchfulness of the breath, and synchronized movement of the body begins to create a more harmonious experience.

When practicing qigong:

- Pay attention.
- Consciously practice with intention.
- Be even more watchful as you continue your practice and watch the breath, know what it is doing. Breathing in, going out, are you controlling it or are you doing a breathless practice? I will teach you to take control of what you can take control of in your life. The rest will sort itself out.
- Synchronize your movement with the breath. If your hands go high up into the air and the exercise has you breathe in, then as you do that be sure those two pieces happen simultaneously. Be mindful and precise in your movement.
- If the breath is held in the lower dantian (lower belly) as the arms reach their high point and then the belly is tightened and then the arms begin to lower and, as they do, the breath is being held or softly released—or in some cases pushed out—then be mindful of that. Pay attention.
- If, in the exercise, the breath is supposed to be released as the arms are moving downward and you are supposed to exhale and move the arms at the same rate of speed so that when your arms get to the bottom of your movement, the breath completes at the same time then try your best to do that.
- If the intention in an exercise is to be slow and relaxed, then be slow and relaxed. If the intention is to push down with some effort and make a sound like "shhhh" while contracting the belly, then pay attention to that.
- I often tell my students that you will get out of qigong what you put into it. If you practice with little attention and cannot even juggle two pieces of the practice then there is no way you will get

out of it the same thing as someone who is juggling five pieces at the same time while being mindful of those five pieces.

- Some practices are simple and you do not have to do much, whereas others require more effort, more attention, and more discipline.

I believe that one of the reasons that qigong can be such a potent practice is that it brings you to the present moment, it brings you—the greater you, the observer in you—to this moment, to your body, to this earth. It helps you to show up; in fact it is a practice of showing up!

This is sometimes called a practice of mindfulness. Being mindful about what you are doing in the moment is essential to breaking the bad habits of yesterday. By bringing this attention, you begin to lay the hidden power of intention upon that attention and then further strengthen that intention with your breath. So if your intention is healing and you are holding that as an intention, the question is how long can you pay attention?

Remember, attention brings energy and, in this case, it brings energy to your intention. If you cease to pay attention, it all falls flat. It takes time to become somewhat masterful with qigong, because it requires a bit of discipline. You may soon, however, find this discipline fun and refreshing!

One of the things that I have always loved best about qigong and martial arts practices is that I cannot focus on my problems and do the exercises at the same time. The exercises require that I show up and set down my life in order to do them correctly and mindfully. I love that. It becomes a moving meditation. Other times it is a still meditation, but even focusing on stillness in the face of resistance requires a particular kind of focus, and I love that.

I have mentioned this at least once or twice in other parts of the book, but learning how to focus your attention and pay attention is a necessary requirement for so many areas of your life. If you train it in qigong you will embody it and take it back with you into your life.

Remember that breath houses chi, so when you breathe that and bring that into your body and being and impregnate that extra energy with intention—the intention for healing, for example—you are working with a potent force. If you mindfully extend that breath and intention throughout your body, you can generate a lot of energy and healing power.

Let's see how some of this works in an actual qigong exercise—you can watch my qigong exercise videos and practice along with me if you like.

## *Qigong Exercise: Cultivating the Force*

- Stand in a horse stance, feet shoulder width apart, knees slightly bent. Be mindful—pay attention.
- Relax your breath, let it just settle. Exhale, setting your intention to relax yourself.
- Circle your palms out away from your belly and reach palms up toward the sky. (Don't worry if you do not get this exactly right; just think through some of these pieces. You can watch the videos later.) As you are performing this motion, take a slow breath in. If you breathe in slowly through the nose you will fill the lower belly first. If you keep breathing slowly, you will then begin to fill your lower lungs and then your upper lungs.
- When your arms reach the highest position, your belly should be full of breath and so should your lungs.
- Now tighten your belly and hold your breath down in your lower belly for a few seconds. Contract your abdominal muscles. Hold it in.
- Let your arms fall and as they do, slowly let your breath out, first through your nose and then through your mouth.
- If you just let all your breath come out through your mouth, you are not holding the chi in. Remember, chi rides on the breath. Chi and oxygen are joined. So if you just let your breath go out of your mouth (try it), you will feel your energy going right out with it. If you keep it and let it out slowly, you will feel more energy from it.
- As you let the breath out, let your arms come down like they are gently pushing down on a cloud. When the exhale finishes, your hands should finish just below the level of your waist. This is an example of synchronizing some of the pieces.
- If it is too difficult to sort this out by reading it in a book, do not fret. Use the video instruction to put the pieces together.

As I mentioned, at eighteen, humans begin to age at a significantly increased rate, in part because the thymus gland begins to shrink. Many qigong masters refer to the thymus gland as a doorway to reversing aging and even to immortality.

One of the main ideas here is not just quantity of life, but quality. The thymus gland is also exponentially important in terms of your immune system, helping you fight off infections including the common cold, lung infections, the flu, and much more.

Your body has potent medicine living right inside of it. The thymus gland houses some pretty potent hormones. It also houses what are called T-lymphocytes, a type of white blood cell involved in cell-mediated immunity. Getting this relatively large sac working for us again is key. If you are a healing practitioner and you desire to help a client expedite their own healing process, help them to turn on their thymus gland.

Chi will flow to wherever you place your attention. Here's a basic qigong exercise to activate the thymus gland.

## Qigong Exercise: Activate the Thymus Gland

- Stand with your feet shoulder-width apart in a natural stance, knees slightly bent. If you are more confident sitting down, then try that position close to the edge of your chair with your spine straight. Standing pose will generate more chi, but if you get dizzy easily, or your legs are not strong enough, then try it seated.
- Lay both your hands on your upper chest below the neck, which is where the thymus gland is located.
- Take three deep breaths and breathe into your lower belly and all the way up to your chest. Hold the intention to wake up and activate your thymus gland.
- After you take the three breaths, relax your breath and simply observe it. No need to control it.
- Now try to relax your hands and arms while still holding them in position on (or hovering above your upper chest.)
- Wait and watch. Five minutes, ten minutes, twenty minutes. The longer you do it, the greater the healing power.

- If someone—a client, for example—is not well and you wish to do this qigong exercise for them in a medical qigong fashion, then you would lay both your hands, one on top of the other, on their upper chest. Stand or sit as comfortably as possible, especially if you want to give them a longer session of ten minutes or more.
- Start with a three- or five-minute round. After the time is up, slowly remove your hands, raising them high up into the air as if you are raising up the chi and expanding it. Then wait for a minute and watch the person's breathing change. Then hold their feet and help them to ground their energy. Have them open and close their fingers and wiggle their toes.
- When practicing on yourself, pay close attention to your throat and the swallowing activity or lack thereof. If you are swallowing one or several times, you are headed in the right direction. If you or your client does not swallow, this could indicate a blockage in chi flow and the length and/or the frequency of the sessions needs to be increased.
- Whether you are practicing on yourself or another person, watch the activity of the blood flow to the neck. You will see the blood flow in the jugular vein taking on a pumping action. Whoever is experiencing that pumping action can feel a medicine pumping through their veins. Eventually this becomes a euphoric experience with major health benefits.

## The Force of Chi

The force of chi has to do with electromagnetism, energy, and therefore electrical charge. It is all around you, and your body is like a battery in that it can take in a charge and hold it. Unlike a battery, you can stretch the amount of charge that you can take in and hold. You must practice gathering chi through the qigong exercises themselves if you want to use this particular type of shortcut to more energy, health, and vitality.

Qigong is a potent practice that is a straight shot to raw, essential, vital energy. It is especially useful when your energy is depleted. If you have developed bad habits, qigong can become the new habit with a different outcome. If you are an injured athlete and want to get back in the game, qigong can help you heal more quickly than anything else I know of. Coupled with the declarations, affirmations, and incantations I have shared with you, qigong can help you generate greater power for yourself.

Once you have developed your chi through qigong practices, you would be wise to do the other exercises such as power walking and power talking over your body before, after, and between your regular qigong practice. If you do not include these mindfulness practices, you will spend what you have gained so quickly that you will most likely not be satisfied with the results.

Typically, people who feel and experience chi the least are people who have the least amount of it. Do not feel bad if you do not feel something mysterious right away or ever. Chi is not much different than blood and oxygen in terms of how you might feel it. You do not have to go out of your body and have a mystical experience to access the deeper wisdom and healing power of qigong.

I was introduced to qigong practice during my hard-style karate martial arts training. I did not know of its healing benefits initially, but I practiced so much during my first three years of training—more than several hours every day—that my hands began to surge with energy. I used that energy to break boards and bricks and I used the chi to protect myself when being struck by an opponent. I also learned eventually to use that chi to heal an injury and I also eventually learned to use those charged hands to heal others.

## Qigong, Jing, Sexual Energy, and Fertility

Until you develop your core—the lower dantian—there can be no surging in the hands. There can be no excess energy, heat, charge, or vitality. The lower belly is depleted, so the sexual energy reserves and therefore overall energy reserves are depleted. With practice this will build up again. Older gentlemen who are well past their teens, twenties, and forties will have the core-essence chi called jing again. This may allow them to become erect again in certain cases and may also enhance fertility as well as enhancing overall energy levels.

Women who regain their chi essence will have more regular periods and less cramping and other complications. Older women who are premenopausal may begin regular periods again. Women who have been struggling with infertility may become pregnant. This is obviously important for those who wish to become pregnant, but jing also enhances vital life force and your ability to heal yourself.

In addition, it also improves your powers of attraction. Where do they come from? The power to attract a friend, a lover, or a new career? No raw essence chi, no jing, no fire, and no passion means you don't have enough life force to attract what you really desire. If you don't have enough life force, you cannot digest your food, manage your stress, or keep your liver and gallbladder functioning properly. Without enough life force, you cannot heal your back, head, and neck pain. Without enough energy, you cannot envision a new business, a new career, or a new master plan for your life.

## Qigong for Better Digestion

If you want to make those bodily systems move then you have to charge that lower belly. All of the qigong exercises that I teach, including the power walking and talking, are designed to gather heat in that belly. When the heat first builds in your belly you might feel uncomfortable. It can feel like a pressure. Remember, the chi wants to build up and, when it does, it then wants to course throughout the body and up the spine.

It is also important to note that there are major lymph nodes in the lower belly, as well as a very large nerve called your vagus nerve. The lower belly is also an epicenter of acupuncture meridians.

If you have eaten a little too much before your qigong practice, you might have some digestion issues. If you have a swollen belly, which many people have, you will feel the pressure of the chi building up inside and it will feel a bit uncomfortable. This is occurring because you have stagnation in your organs related to digestion—stomach, small intestine, liver, gall bladder, large intestine, etc.

But if you practice and pace yourself, you will begin to purge some of that stagnation. You will have better bowel movements. If your belly is swollen you might (sometimes for some people) initially have diarrhea, but do not be concerned. That is just your body cleaning things out, and things will normalize. In rare instances, people vomit, but only if their body has become too toxic. This is more common in cancer patients and is a way for the body to detoxify.

## Qigong and Weight Loss

People who exercise have a higher metabolism rate, so they burn calories more quickly. Qigong practice will increase your internal heat and burn more calories if you are overweight. There are certain exercises that are more effective for increasing metabolism, but this style of qigong helps balance hormones and organ systems so that you can stabilize your weight. The emphasis is not only on the physical practice but also on your emotional well-being. Getting control over your thoughts and feelings is essential when it comes to losing weight.

In this book, I have given you exercises to think and speak over your body. This is going to help you get into the right mindset. Remember that thoughts produce emotions and therefore moods. You need to deal with these thoughts and their representatives called words, and you need to also take charge of your moods and emotions.

If you were to begin doing that, your diet would look different, you would be attracted to different foods, and your metabolism would be faster because of the practice. This is about changing your lifestyle, not about losing ten pounds in one day or one week. When you change your lifestyle and your habits, your body will follow suit. In this way, qigong practice has the ability to promote weight loss from a variety of perspectives.

Simultaneously, because qigong focuses on balancing bodily functions, someone who needs to gain weight could be practicing the same exercises as someone who needs to lose weight, and both could accomplish their goals. This is often possible through qigong practice, although, in some cases, there are very specific practices for one outcome versus another.

## Medical Qigong

I mentioned that after a few years of training in qigong, my hands began to surge with energy and they would get very hot. I was studying different disciplines in addition to my martial arts and qigong training, among them massage and medical qigong healing practices.

I began directing my mind and my hands toward other people with the intention of healing, and profound things began to occur. I will share with you some of my earlier experiences. Remember that medical qigong is a primary form of Oriental medicine. It is the father of the more modern acupuncture. It is one of the four branches of Oriental medicine that include medical qigong, acupuncture, massage, and herbs. After thirty years of qigong practice, I am now a medical qigong master and teach qigong and medical qigong workshops around the country. I combine qigong education for personal healing and development with the practice of extending healing to others.

The force of chi can be gathered and can be run through you. The more you call to it (so to speak), the more it comes. You can call it for yourself and you can also call it for others. When you call it for others, it still has to come through you, so you get the chi too. It is true that facilitating healing for others can drain you initially, but over the hours, days, and weeks you will become stronger and stronger. If I were to go to the gym tonight and lift weights I would be tired afterwards. With rest, good nutrition, and return visits to the gym, though, my body would become stronger. You do not get stronger overnight, but over a period of time. Medical qigong practices follow those same principles. You will not get stronger overnight but over a period of time as you follow a regimen of practice, rest, and practice.

This section is for those who are curious and for those who are interested in facilitating healing for others as many of my current students are. Many of my students are acupuncturists, massage therapists, chiropractors, nurses, physical therapists, medical doctors, counselors, etc.

If you wish to facilitate healing for others, qigong is a valuable skill. Many healers, whether they are doctors, therapists, acupuncturists, nurses, or other practitioners, are giving, giving, giving all the time and do not have a way to refuel themselves. Refueling yourself through qigong practice is a great way to increase longevity, improve the effectiveness of your treatments, and keep you nourished and on top of your game.

As a medical qigong practitioner, how might you help another person's body to heal? Medical qigong helps restore the flow of chi in, around and through the body, so you are helping your client's body to heal itself.

## Medical Qigong Healing Case Studies

Here are examples of healings I have facilitated in my private practice. These case studies demonstrate the range of qigong healing potential across space and species.

*Family and Friends*

During the early years of my career, I was doing bodywork and offering clothed massage, deep tissue massage, and some basic energy work to family and friends. Then something began to shift for me. I would get close to someone to work on them and their body would react as if to an electrical field. Their body would jump or start to undulate as if a wave of energy was passing through them. People would often go into states of REM (rapid eye movements associated with deeper states of sleep). They would wake up very refreshed and often pain-free or healed of some other problem.

*Dogs*

I had a dog who had parasitic worms; they were several inches long and there were too many to count every time she defecated. I was working as a supervisor in a hospital at the time and could not take my dog to the vet's until the following morning. When I was at work I felt really bad for my dog. I had the thought "Why can't I just use my psychic power to kill these parasites?" I began trying immediately. When I returned home after my shift I expected my apartment and my porch to be a disaster, but it wasn't. I then expected my dog would go outside and have a wet stool filled with worms. She went out and had a normal stool.

I called the vet the next morning and asked him if she could have pooped them out. He said, "Absolutely not, bring in a stool sample." I brought in a stool sample and he called and said, "You must have been mistaken because there is no trace of microscopic organisms here." I was blown away. I wondered, "Could I have possibly done this?"

Then my roommate had a dog with a bone lodged in his intestines. My roommate had to follow this dog around with a baggie and the vet said that if his dog did not pass the bone in the next twenty-four hours, the dog would have to go in for emergency surgery in the morning. We had x-rays and I was able to observe the bone. I practiced using my mind to dissolve the energy of the bone. The next morning an x-ray was taken to determine where the bone was lodged, for it had not passed through the dog yet. There was no trace of the bone. The vet said that my roommate must have missed it in the dog's stool, but the dog never pooped.

Another dog had several tumors on her legs. She was scheduled for surgery the following morning. My client brought the dog to me, then sat in the van outside my office. I went out and scanned the dog and began to smooth out her chi. Her chi was rough and bumpy—that is what it felt like. I visualized the tumors dissolving and worked with the energy to reshape the molecular structure almost as if I were working with clay. The next morning the tumors were all gone. The surgery was canceled, and the tumors did not return.

*Baby Boy*

I saw a baby boy with holes in his heart (like Swiss cheese, according to his doctors). They said he needed open-heart surgery when he turned four months old. He arrived at my office with an oxygen tank in tow. You could not see his neck because he constantly shrugged and rolled his neck like he was writhing in pain. I had facilitated a healing for one of his relatives who had a severe case of shingles. Her shingles were quite obvious and significant. Her eye and face were severely swollen and she could not open her right eye. After two treatments, the shingles disappeared. She soon brought in this new baby to see if he too could have a healing.

After four months of weekly treatments, the baby boy was taken in for a pre-op for his open-heart surgery. To the doctor's disbelief, the boy's heart was healed. All of the holes in the heart, including one significant hole, had sealed up. The doctor said that the baby had had a miracle healing. When you understand yourself, your body, your energy field, your emotions, etc., it becomes that much easier to help others heal themselves.

*Bacteria*

I performed an experiment for my final in a molecular and cellular biology lab class at the University of Colorado at Boulder in which I placed E. Coli on a bacterial dish and I sent my mind to that dish to eradicate the bacteria. I was able to perform this experiment because of Larry Dossey, M.D.'s book *The Power of Prayer*. That book included many such experiments done by researchers demonstrating the power of the mind and its influence over energy and matter. I was able to achieve a significant decrease in the number of bacteria on that plate.

*Rabbit*

I had a student with me during a program and her daughter called in a state of hysteria. She was traveling to the emergency vet hospital because her rabbit's eye was protruding from its head due to some sort of inflammation. I immediately began sending healing thoughts and energy to the daughter and the rabbit. By the time the daughter arrived at the emergency room, which was about sixty minutes away, the rabbit was already healed. The vet saw no signs of any problem and nothing of that nature occurred with the rabbit again.

*Female Client with Large Cyst*

A woman I had met at one of my workshops called me for a long-distance healing. She had some type of large growth in her neck the size of a tennis ball. The doctors said that if it wasn't dissolved by morning they would need to surgically remove it. It was not responding to antibiotics. I sensed this woman's energetic field. I began to speak to certain things I saw going on and I began to work with that energy and influence it. By morning the swelling had disappeared. Her white blood counts returned to normal and she was given a clean bill of health.

*Male Client with Pain*

A college football player told me he had had a third surgery on his knee. He said he was on pain meds, but they were not working. He was a very large, rough and tumble kind of guy, but he was in tears. I began working on him and within minutes the pain was more tolerable. After a couple of treatments, he was mostly pain-free and very grateful.

*Male Client with High Blood Pressure*

A gentleman came in with chronic high blood pressure. His medication was keeping things at bay, but the pressure on multiple levels continued to be an issue. After two or three treatments, his blood pressure was significantly lower and—under his doctor's supervision—he was able to go off the medication.

*Female Client with Exhaustion*

A woman came into to my office complaining of adrenal burnout, fatigue, and lethargy. I charged her energy field over the course of several sessions. From day one she said, "I can tell you are not working on my body. I feel like I am floating on the table." She said, "I thought this would be like acupuncture, I know it is related but this is something different." After building up her chi—in this case her raw base chi or jing—she was full of energy again and able to return to her passions.

*Female Client with Infection*

One client was concerned about a medical test that was showing some infection. She had issues with a relationship and was challenged as well by a recent divorce. I called it all out on the table and asked her to speak to it. After she spoke to it, I spoke to it and gave one, two, or three examples of how she might begin speaking to it. I did not just say that I had read a book about this kind of thing and this is what it said. I spoke to her energy while I was teaching her how to do it.

She kept saying things like "Well how am I going to do that?" and "How many times will it take?" and so on. What I made her aware of was that I was doing it and she was following along and therefore helping me do it, right then and there. The next day she had the same test again and she ended up with very different test results. Needless to say, she was very happy about the results. She had learned in this private training session just how powerful her mind is. Granted, I helped her, but she followed along and got to see the results of the practice.

After she spoke to her story, I called out some key hidden phrases that were hiding from her awareness, but were right there in the energy field and easy for me to see. I said, "You might try speaking to that story just like this," and I went on a run of primary thinking, just like I have taught you how to do. I spoke over her body as if it was mine; I spoke over her relationships as if they were mine with a very empowered attitude. I heard her sigh on the phone; I could tell she was shifting into a different state. Very quickly, within twenty-four hours, several things shifted for her, not just the test results, but other obvious shifts as well.

## Qigong Healing and Coaching—How it Works

Directing chi when you understand it better can be done from a distance and can be done with many different techniques. Awareness and intuition play major roles in your skills as a healer. The more skilled you are at working with yourself and the force itself, the more skilled you will be in working with others in conjunction with that force.

These days, I often work with people over the telephone or via Skype. In such cases, I obviously can't lay my hands on them, touch this point or that point, massage this or that shoulder. Yet the healing works! The energy holds the story and it is programmed by the mind and the emotions. It then influences the physical body.

So if you wish to heal the physical body, you might be wise to focus on the energy, the hidden stories and tapes, and you might be wise to reprogram the energy. You can begin that practice by power walking around the room, power walking down the street and using primary thinking where you talk over that noise in your head or that disbelief rambling around in your mind.

When I work with people privately, we cut to the chase and get right to business. I do not counsel people. I help them see what they want to see but maybe are afraid to deal with and then we deal with it very quickly by reprogramming the energy. When the energy shifts, the person feels different and then they have the "ah ha" and see things differently. This approach is unlike most psychology practices. It is similar to life coaching, but with one key difference—the focus is on the energetic nature of the person.

We are—literally—all connected. If a client chooses to join me on the phone, for example, and speak to an issue, that issue is brought into awareness. If a person doesn't know how to effectively deal with those thoughts, those emotions, and the energy they create, then that person is on that roller coaster with no way of getting off the ride. When I work with people in that predicament, I bring a confidence because of the qigong practices and what I have come to know as the process of how our mind-body-soul works. I will speak to the energy and I tell it—the energy—a different story. I, in essence, give it a different command. Program it anew.

This can be done silently or out loud. It can be done with an obvious technique, such as the extension of a hand, or a not so obvious technique, during which I work with the energy only on the level of my mind. Because of the client's intention to join me in healing, their defenses and their guard will rest to some degree. In that rest, it is as if the client says, "Go ahead and take the wheel for a moment of time." In that moment, I take the wheel and I speak to the energy; I communicate with it and I do it with confidence. The energy will always respond. Some people's energy is much thicker than others and therefore less willing to move, but even in such cases the energy will move eventually. For the client, this process brings about a healing experience and a deeper understanding of who they are and what their energetic makeup is.

During silent work, the same kind of reprogramming happens. If you know how to connect with that force and you lay your intention upon it and speak to it or just hold a thought to it and begin to work with the energy of it, shifts will occur. It takes practice and that takes time, but I think it is usually super fun and very empowering. Not always fun, not always easy, sometimes a bit intimidating if you are trying to do it on your own, but in time it will become easier and easier.

For more information on becoming a qigong instructor and coach as well as a medical qigong healing practitioner, check out the certification page on our website.

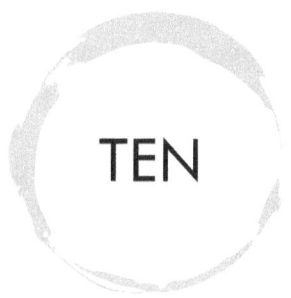

# TEN

# CLEANSING THE EMOTIONAL PAIN BODY

---

"Rather than being your thoughts and emotions, be the awareness behind them." Eckhart Tolle

---

Eckhart Tolle is a modern spiritual teacher and the author of the best-selling book, *A New Earth: Awakening to your Life's Purpose.* In this book, Tolle refers to something he calls the pain body. The pain body is not a new concept—masters of meditation, yoga, and qigong have referred to it as the emotional body for centuries.

You might want to add *A New Earth* to your reading list (Oprah put it on hers!). Tolle helps readers gain an awareness of this subtle and elusive aspect of themselves as well as an understanding of the power of observation, meditation, and awareness.

Because many masters refer to this energy as the emotional body and Tolle calls it the pain body, I am combining the terms here to bring awareness to the whole dynamic. Here are some qigong exercises to bring healing to the emotional pain body.

In the last chapter, I referred to the emotional pain body as energy when I said that I speak to the energy in my private work with people. Whether I am coaching or offering a medical qigong treatment, I am communicating with that energy. I also made the point that I do not counsel people—I speak directly to the energy and help them reprogram it. This can be done out loud, perhaps using primary thinking to speak over someone's internal dialogue, which is often hidden and is held energetically. This energy that I speak to has a lot to do with the emotional pain body.

The emotional pain body houses memories from your consciously remembered past as well as all of your unconscious memory—that of all your past—including pre-birth. You can think in terms of the emotional pain body containing information gathered while you were in the womb or—if you are Buddhist (for example)—you might think in terms of information from any and all previous incarnations. This subtle, invisible (to most) energy field or pain body goes with you wherever you go, and, for most people, it is largely unhealed, leading to both mental and physical disease as well as other life challenges.

The emotional pain body is part of the mind and remains mostly subconscious, which means you are largely unaware of its content. Despite that fact, your actions, inactions, reactions, addictions, and fears are driven by the information contained within the emotional pain body. (Take a deep breath. This part of the mind does not like to be observed out in the open and it does not like change, so try to stay with me.)

Your negative reactions to people, places, things, and events, whether they manifest as anger, greed, jealousy, anxiety, self-hatred, self-doubt, and/or depression or fear, are all hidden to some degree or another in this emotional body. In fact, they are often stuffed in there. Typically, your emotions rise into your awareness when you emotionally react to someone or to some event. Somebody or some event happens—someone cuts you off in traffic, comes home late, bothers you at work, etc. The outer stimulus provokes you, and your feelings of resistance to that outer stimulus cause unwanted emotions to rise. These old unwanted emotions can be stressful and many of us eat sweets or eat to excess, drink alcohol, smoke cigarettes, chew gum, take medications, bite our nails, gossip, stare blankly at the television, etc., to avoid them. People do all of these things and more in an attempt to repress, suppress, stuff down whatever is rising into their awareness. This, of course, causes pain, illness, disease, and more life challenges.

Awareness is a key point of focus for meditation, yoga, qigong, and many martial arts teachers. Awareness is often referred to as the eternal flame, which has the ability to dissolve whatever it observes. In general, then, awareness is meditation, awareness is observation, awareness is the remedy.

Meditation, in general terms, means awareness without judgment. This type of practice leads to the kind of alchemy referenced throughout the book, and through which you can learn to sit and observe and stare, laying attention upon anger, for example, burning it in the cauldron of the lower dantian and turning it into metaphorical gold. Some people practice seated meditation, others martial arts meditation, some lie down, and some stand like a tree. I find standing like a tree to be a particularly potent form of meditation.

Qigong practice can dissolve the emotional pain body. It allows you to burn through it (relatively) quickly. Not all forms of qigong are designed to do this in the same way, but the forms I teach focus on this objective. The different movement and stillness practices, the breath control, and/or the breath observation etc., are all designed to promote emotional purification.

This emotional cleansing may not seem to be emotional at all, any more than someone running up a mountain into their thirteenth mile of a 26-mile marathon would say "I got to the thirteenth mile and I got really emotional for a minute." That may happen to some people, but most can't breathe, have cramps, and feel pain.

Qigong practice is similar to running a race. You can walk it, jog it, run it, sprint it, slow it down, etc. You can use similar approaches to get through the emotional pain body without ever leaving your living room. I will teach you one of my favorite qigong purification exercises that will allow you to purify and detox this emotional pain body.

## The Emotional Pain Body

The emotional pain body does not like attention; it likes habit and distraction and dissipation of energy. You could say that it has a mind of its own. Some psychologists and spiritual teachers refer to it as ego—I do too.

Scientists are discovering that the human gut is a kind of second brain. It seems the gut—the lower dantian in Chinese medicine—does more than digest food. It has its own programming. Guess where your reactions live.

Think about it. When you give up your energy to bad habits—heavy drinking, too much sex, too much foul language, too many dysfunctional relationships, smoking, excess negative thinking, excess negative speech, etc.—you deplete yourself of vital life force. If you've read this far, that should be a no-brainer.

What may not be as obvious, though, is that you are trying to dissipate your attention and awareness of your pain. When you have pain, you would more often than not rather it go away. Learning to be with your pain—physically, emotionally, and mentally—as well as dissipate it and transmute it—is a skill. Gathering energy to yourself and then using that energy to purify the emotional pain body requires practice.

The ancient alchemists (see CHAPTER FIVE: THE ALCHEMIST) saw the lower belly as a cooking pot where the lower emotions like anger, greed, jealousy, etc. are burned. Deal with your pain body effectively and your level of inner peace over time increases exponentially because as you purify this pain, you purify yourself and cleanse yourself of the past.

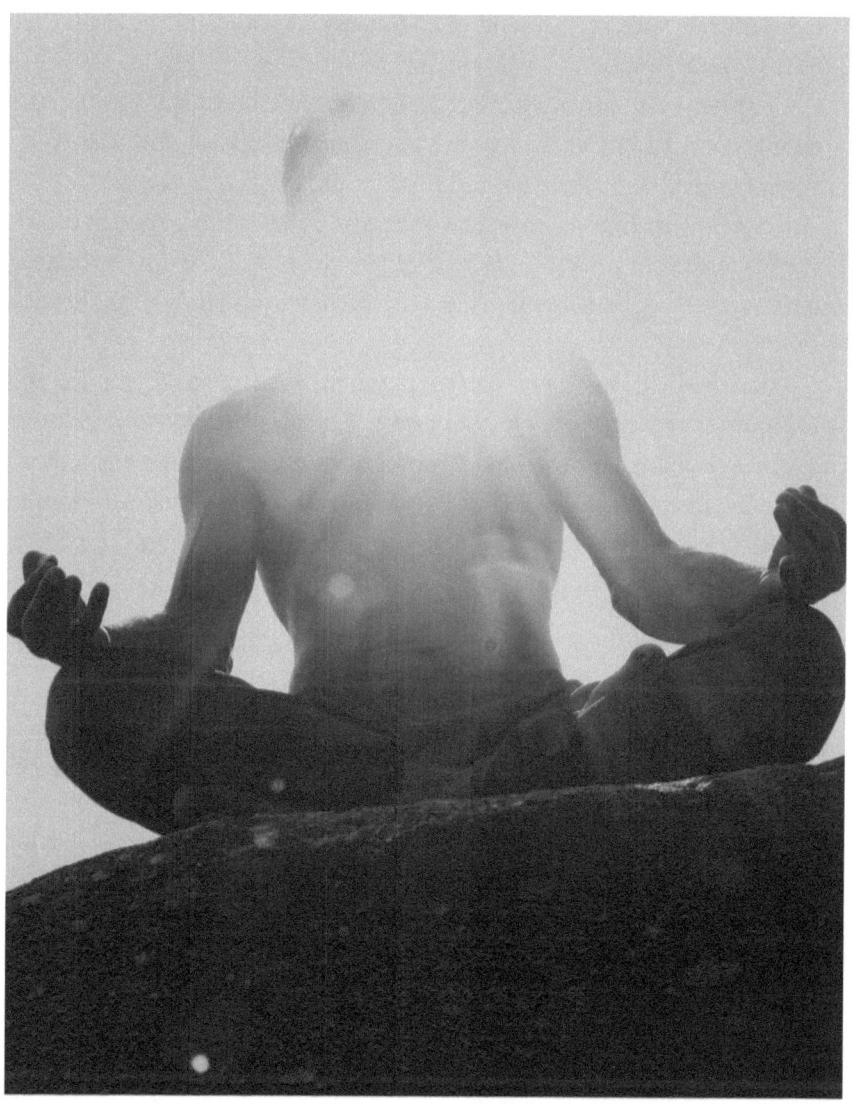

*Photo by: Lisa Siciliano*

Where is the past? Without you, it may not exist. With you and with the thoughts you hold about it, the past can cause incredible pain. Without your past pain, you would be joyful and free because trauma and past and future fear would be absent. It is also important to note that in such states, you would not have the same level of toxicity in your body, and toxicity causes physical disease.

What you eat is important. Much of the food you buy in the supermarket contains agricultural and other poisons. In addition, your body has to deal with toxic air and toxic water.

Masters teach that outer reality is created by your inner state of mind. If they're correct, as you clean up your inner state of mind and its associated emotions, you will be helping to clean up the environment you share with others.

Emotional disease often causes physical disease, so if you change your emotional state—which is not easy, but it is doable—you remove the source of many, many forms of physical disease. I include any and all injuries in this chain of causation, because emotional unrest also results in injuries. Emotional unrest is your unfinished business, and until you finish it, it will keep running your life.

## Qigong Exercise: Standing Tree Meditation

All of the qigong exercises I teach will deal with the emotional pain body. They will set it on fire, cleanse it, clear it, and purge it, and this will detoxify your cells, organs, and tissues, even down to the cellular blueprint called DNA. Having said that, I want to introduce you to a potent qigong exercise that is not only one of my favorites, but is easily conveyed in writing.

It is called standing tree meditation. Stand with your feet shoulder width apart and bend your knees slightly. Your eyes can remain open, but be sure to use a steady, relaxed gaze rather than looking all around the room. If you do the meditation with your eyes closed, you will gather even more subtle energy.

Think of your emotional pain body as your nervous system and all of its previous programming. It is filled with resistance, and resistance blocks flow and causes pain and disease. If the lymph stops flowing well, you can get cancer. If the blood stops flowing well, you can get heart disease. If the acupuncture meridians do not flow well, you can have organ issues. If you have organ issues, you can have multiple issues in your joints, tissues, etc. For example, a stagnant liver can lead to pain in the right shoulder. A stagnant stomach can cause migraines, and so on.

- Set a timer for 5, 10, or 15 minutes to start.
- Once the timer is set, stand in the pose. Arms are simply down at your side.
- The rules of the practice are:
    o Do not move.
    o Do not scratch.
    o Do not readjust except for a very simple realignment in the beginning as you straighten your spine.
    o Be still.
- It does not matter what you think—initially do not worry about it.
- The main thing is to be still and not move.
- Observe your body.
- Initially, your mind will go here and there; come back and remind yourself of what you are doing so that you do not fall asleep and you do not move.

During every minute you stand like this, you are gathering energy to yourself that you usually spend moving and looking around the room and so on. It may take years of practice before your mind gets quiet. I don't mean sleepy, I mean quiet, and there is a difference.

But don't worry about any of that. Set the timer and do your best. Increase the length of time you spend doing the meditation as well as how often you do it every month. It will change you from the inside out in subtle but profound ways. Sixty minutes would be considered an intermediate practice and four hours an advanced practice.

As you practice tree meditation, notice when you swallow (or don't). Also, notice the difference in your overall sense of well-being afterwards. If you were angry, depressed, or anxious when you started, notice how the meditation changes the energy dynamic. Notice that once the energy dynamic shifts, so does your mood. Notice that with the shift of your mood, your thoughts about yourself, about life, and about tomorrow change.

The emotional pain body is closely associated with your intellect or mental body. As you alchemize the second chakra energy—pain-body-related information—you may also begin to purify the mental body, which is closely associated with second chakra energy. The mental body is related to the third chakra and the solar plexus, also known as your power center.

If you can successfully clear some of this second and third chakra stagnation, you may come into what Tolle and other master teachers refer to as "the moment." You are no longer future-focused and anxious; you are no longer focused on your past and depressed. For a moment, you are free. Tolle likes to use the word "being" to describe this place of inner quiet, solitude, and presence.

## No Mind

Being in the moment is another way of saying that you are in a state of "no mind," a concept common in qigong, martial arts, and meditation training. No mind is not a brainless state. It is not being brain dead, repressed, lethargic, or high on some drug. No mind is a state of mind that is relaxed, present and clear. Some martial arts masters can enter this state even during combat; I have experienced it myself. You discover it when the emotional pain body is quiet—not dormant, not hidden in unawareness— but either transcended for a moment or purified.

You can rise above your fear in a moment to become centered (if you have the skill) and face five other opponents with swords, for example. Or you can show up to your full-contact Karate tournament and—even though you are afraid—rise above that fear and/or center yourself so that your mind is clear and you can do what you need to do.

Rising above your fear in a moment and/or dropping into your center is a very useful skill that comes with training. Managing your mind and your breath allows you to manage your emotions. For a police officer driving at high rates of speed trying to catch bad guys, a person giving a speech in front of a large audience, or a student taking a final exam, this skill comes in handy. There are thousands of places and situations this skill is useful, and yet it was not taught in any conventional school I ever attended.

This is changing, though. Some schools are incorporating mindfulness practice into their schedules to help students de-stress and give their brains a break. This improves attention spans and creates a more relaxed atmosphere.

No mind is also a mind state that is achieved over the course of a well-lived lifetime by masters of various disciplines. Buddhists suggest that it takes many lifetimes of practice to achieve such a state. In the context of healing and/or seeking enlightenment, it is a state of presence and deep, undisturbed awareness; a state of inner peace and tranquility.

Many people try to shortcut to these mysterious or mystical states. Although I agree that you should seek shortcuts or life hacks, you're unlikely to achieve the healing and the inner peace from which greater health and vitality can arise without effort.

The question is, how badly do you want to change, heal, and transform yourself? I wasn't drawn to healing myself and bettering my life because I was bored and did not have anything to do on Friday night—it was because I was in pain. It was because I was in a lot of pain and my life was—in general—not the life I wanted to be living. There were a lot of people, situations, and dynamics that I wanted to change. I tried shifting them, healing them, fixing them, counseling them, avoiding them, etc., but none of it worked. So I changed myself from the inside out.

When someone or something internal or external comes into your world and causes you upset that manifests as depression, repression, negative emotion, anger, greed, sadness, rage, grief, etc., you know your emotional pain body is active. It has been lit up. Some people try to spiritualize themselves and their lives and hide from others because they think, "other people are so crazy," and other similar thoughts.

Again, life is a mirror. If you do not like what you are seeing in your mirror, you can hide for a while, but be sure to do something about your energy, your emotional pain body, because if you are seeing outer challenges and you are having internal reactions to those challenges, your emotional pain body is lit up. If your emotional pain body keeps lighting up, you need to clean it up to achieve the peace of mind that comes with no mind.

Find mental and emotional clarity and the physical healing will come. As happiness and inner peace come too, you will see your outer world of circumstances, people, places, and events begin to calm down, chill, improve. When things ramp up again and the inner calm goes away, come back to the practice.

This is why I offer qigong as a lifestyle and even a career path. This world is not built for healing now—you have to work for it and design your life in such a way that healing becomes a priority. If you don't do that in some way in your life through qigong or another pursuit such as yoga, martial arts, art, writing, acting, or something else, then what you seek will more than likely elude you forever while you deplete yourself chasing it. In order to achieve something worthwhile, you typically have to get centered and make an educated, consistent effort.

You are a result of your habits. We are all creatures of habit, but some habits will reveal great things about us and other habits will make us feel anything but great.

If you make qigong a habit—perhaps you teach it to others or adopt it as part of your new lifestyle—then that habit will bring certain results. Those results include healing, self-improvement, confidence, greater vitality, and increased longevity, to name only a few. You might even build a career out of it as I have. The alternative medicine business is a billion-dollar affair. People are willing to pay way more than your ten or twenty or even fifty dollars an hour for whatever hourly work you are currently doing.

If you adopt this as a career path, qigong and medical qigong are forms of schooling and training that can help you have your cake and eat it too. I believe that as you give to others, life gives back to you. I have proved that to myself, time and time again. Qigong practices, teaching qigong, and offering medical qigong healing are all good karma for me and for the world around me.

That is what I wish to share with you. A few Caucasian folks have forged this path here in the West, and I am on the front end of that with them and I believe many more will follow. This work is not limited to Asian masters or long-time yogis, although we can learn from them. Our school provides a structured curriculum that includes much of that learning.

When you are in physical pain, practice. Be mindful, breathe, do something about that injury—don't just sit there feeling sorry for yourself.

When you are in pain emotionally, breathe, take charge, go for a walk, and reprogram your mind, your body, and your life. When your emotional pain body is lit up like a Christmas tree, go hide from your friends and family for a while and do a qigong routine. When you are feeling nervous because of your upcoming exam or your speech before a crowd of fifty people, go practice a short qigong routine and clear your breath, your body, and your mind. If and when you feel unmotivated to do it on your own, turn me on—I will come to your house via an Internet video and help you practice! Every time you practice qigong, you are tapping into a higher power, but you have to practice it.

## Common Cold

So many people—most of us, in fact—want to be somewhere better than they are right now. Rather than worrying about that, though, do something, namely qigong, today that is going to make a difference today and thirty days from now. If you have a cold creeping up on you and you understand some of the power walking and power talking qigong practices I gave you earlier, you can stop the cold in its tracks. It's easier at that stage than if you let it go into full effect. Colds and flus are not just about bacteria and viruses, they are related to emotions.

Too many emotions, too much stress creates a weakened immune system. The bigger picture is that a weakened immune system makes you susceptible to bacteria and viruses. The best defense is always a good offense, so always try to stay ahead of the game with your health—build it up when you're feeling healthy and energized. When you're not on top of your game, get on it as soon as you realize that. If you know you have been stressed and you know you have not been practicing but you also know you are getting sick, you still have a chance to not be sick. Practice qigong.

A lot of people realize they are getting sick, but they will still not practice qigong because they want to be sick. They do not want to have the physical effects of the sickness but they do want the attention they are going to get. They do want to have the day off from work. They do want to blame another family member for getting them sick. Human beings who are in pain and/or wrestling with the emotional pain body are not totally sane or thinking clearly.

There are more empowered ways to get what you want than getting sick. If you're already sick, though, do not fret. Take steps to reclaim your power. That power is in your choice, your breath, exercising your mind, exercising your power of attention and intention. If you choose lazy as your habit, you will live the results of lazy. If you practice your qigong practices, you will reap the results of those practices. If your habit is to blame others, you might piss them off, but you will make yourself sick. When you realize it is not worth it, you might practice qigong or go for a power walk and power talk instead.

Do your colds and flus have to do with your emotional pain body? Yes, they do.

Do they have to do with your pent up emotions? Yes, they do.

Do they have to do with your attitude toward yourself and toward your life? Yes, they do?

Do they have to do with your relationships both at home and at work? Yes, they do.

When you have a cold or a flu, is it because the kids at school have been sick or the people at the hospital have been sick? In part, perhaps, but the bigger picture is, did you lose your center, did you react, did you overreact, did their actions or nonactions stress you out, upset you? If they did, then consider the possibility that your upset might be the bigger cause of your sickness.

Next time someone is sick in your world, try not to take that sickness personally and emotionally. Watch what happens. In an advanced practice, everyone around you can be sick, and despite the poison floating through the air, you will be unaffected.

In order to be sick, you have to say yes to being sick. You have to say yes to the pathogen and you have to say yes to the sickness and you have to say yes to joining someone else in sickness and you have to want it for some reason. It is not about fighting against it either, because that which you resist persists. It is about rising above it. Walk your walk, talk your power talk over your own water and your own immune system and if the person you are with wants sickness and proclaims it to be their right, they are correct, it is. You, however, do not have to join them in that process unless you want to.

Have you ever noticed how many older married couples compete for who is more sick? Ever been to a dinner party at which you took the time to listen to people talking with each other, or, more specifically, talking to themselves pretending to talk to each other?

In such conversations, you will hear people talking about all their health problems. One is talking loud and so the other talks louder and both are vying for the most attention. If this is ever you, you might want to stop making yourself more and more sick. If it is not, observe these people and simply try to have compassion for where they are in their journey. If someone pins you down and begins to lay into you about how sick they are, trying (unconsciously) to guilt trip you into feeling sorry for them so that two days later you will join them in that sickness, you might want to mindfully practice compassion or you might find yourself sick too.

While they are going off on their story, just try to have compassion; hold the thought of compassion in your heart. If you were angered by the conversation, go talk yourself into a compassionate state.

Do not feel sorry. Do not feel guilty. Do not try to fix people. Just have compassion. In my work, I call it a place of being and that place of being is one of compassionate strength. It takes personal practice to achieve that place of compassionate strength, which is a place of no mind (meaning no worry, no reaction, no judgment). It is attainable over time—with regular practice, you will be able to access it more and more. It doesn't mean you do not feel the pain or the worry or the hurt, but you rise above it, observe it, and meditate on it from above until it begins to dissolve.

## Fear, Anxiety, Depression

When fear is building and you are emotionally distraught, your emotional pain body is lit up and your mind is going haywire, which is the opposite of no mind. Sometimes no mind is also referred to as clear mind. Rather than trying to figure things out, stop, pause, practice, clear your head, and, when your mind is clearer, go back to your life. A confused mind will always breed confusing experiences. Fearful mind will always breed scary experiences. People who have anxiety, for example, are breeding that anxiety without realizing that they are. They are obsessed with what they feel in that moment.

I understand and am not judging, because I spent the first thirty years of my life in that state. Remember, though, that thoughts give rise to emotions through internal messengers like peptides and hormones and those emotions seem to have a life of their own. If you focus on the emotions in such a way as to believe that they are attacking you from the outside, then you give away your power and you will breed even more fear and anxiety.

On the other hand, if you interrupt the cycles of anxiety and/or depression with qigong and qigong breathing practice, then you can take charge of the situation. You are automatically going from being a victim of something to taking charge of that something. You then interrupt the thinking process that produced the emotion in the first place. You then begin to change the blood chemistry, and if you practice enough, you will hit a tipping point and change your mood. Once you change your mood, you will wonder what it was that you were ever afraid of in the first place.

If you are addicted to anxiety and/or depression, you will likely (typically unconsciously) begin thinking the exact same thoughts that caused you anxiety or depression, and very soon your blood will respond accordingly. Before long, your anxiety or depression will be back.

Knowing you have a choice is essential. Making a wiser choice is also essential. Over time, knowing that you are not what you feel, that what you feel is biochemistry and energetic in nature and that you have the power to change it will be incredibly healing and freeing for you. You will not achieve no mind, no reaction, no worry in one day, but in one day you can catch a glimpse of it and over time it will last longer and longer. Qigong gives you a means to do this.

## When and How Often to Practice

I think that twenty minutes a day is a great base to shoot for, which is why I offer a handful of qigong videos that will take you through mini routines. As you build up and are ready for a full qigong class you can combine three twenty-minute videos or try out one of our sixty-minute training sessions live or online. If you practice the core qigong exercises taught to you through our video library and through live workshops and you couple that training with power walking and power talking, you are going to be a force of energy.

If you take it further and become one of our certified qigong instructors, you are going to not only heal yourself but others too! If you are an acupuncturist, massage therapist or other health care provider, teaching a qigong class to your clients and your community is a great way to boost your business. Medical qigong healing will also take your current healing modalities to an even higher level of healing.

## Insomnia

Exercises that involve more movement and more breath are better done in the morning or during the day rather than right before bed. In the evening, a practice like standing tree meditation can help you calm down and get a good night's sleep.

But only after a good practice! Sleep issues like insomnia are an issue because you do not have enough energy. That's right—if you do not have enough energy, you will not be able to get a good night's rest. The body needs subtle vital energy to go into deeper states of sleep. So practice a more vigorous qigong exercise in the morning, afternoon, or even early evening, but then do a standing tree meditation before going to bed. Instructions for enhanced standing tree meditation can be found at the end of this chapter. When you do enhanced standing tree meditation before bed, however, leave out the breath of fire.

## Physical, Mental, and Emotional Disease

Physical, mental, and emotional disease, discomfort, and associated suffering are not necessary. You have the ability to make a difference and cleanse your body, your emotions, and your mind. Resistance, stagnation, and sludge in the physical and emotional body lead to pain and discomfort as well as disease. Negative feelings like frustration, fear, anxiety, depression, pain, and the like can be breathed away. When you couple focused thought (intention) with a complementary body posture and a focused breath, your ability to make a difference in your personal mental, emotional, and physical experience increases exponentially.

Sometimes you can reprogram thoughts and use primary thinking, but sometimes you cannot even get your mind around it and what you need to do is sprint up a mountain. If you could sprint up a mountain it would make all the difference in terms of how you feel, but maybe you cannot physically do that. This next exercise will give you the benefit of sprinting up a mountain and heal your pain body at the same time.

Even if you are someone who likes to sprint up mountains, go right ahead and do it five times and when you cannot do it again, try this exercise. If you are an athlete who is injured, try this exercise. If you are tired and feel depressed or anxious, try this exercise. If something is pushing up into your awareness like anger, greed or jealously and you would rather have inner peace, try this exercise. Back pain? Try this exercise. This exercise has many benefits and can be adapted to your personal situation.

As you do this exercise, think in terms of cleansing and purifying yourself, your pain body, your nervous system, and your past.

### Qigong Exercise: Enhanced Tree Meditation and Breath of Fire

- Stand in tree meditation—natural stance, feet shoulder width apart, knees slightly bent.
- Now to make this an enhanced tree meditation, raise your arms high to the sky.
- If you have shoulder problems and can only raise one arm, raise one arm.
- Now, with attitude, focus up!
- Wake up, yes, but also think up toward the sky.
- Arms to the sky, hands face each other. Freeze.
- Eyes gaze upward.
- Begin a short inhale through the nose only. It goes in and to the belly.
- Then it goes out through the nose only and the belly lowers.
- Try it again.
- Increase the speed of your breath (unless you're doing this practice before bed).

- To do the advanced practice, the breath would be very rapid. To begin with, though, just breathe in and out, in and out, slow and easy.
- To go faster with this breath, you must work through it. Most people cannot run fast and long without practice; working with this breath is analogous to running.
- Once you have a good rhythm, go more quickly.
- Relax your shoulders and your chest as much as possible.

In this somewhat advanced practice (it is an even more advanced practice if you do it for a half hour or more), you want to burn up resistance in the pain body. If you breathe and hold this pose, you will begin to feel the burn. The burn and the pain you feel in your shoulders and elsewhere are the resistance to the chi flow; that is your pain body. When the chi begins to flow there, the pain will dissolve. Until then, it will build and often feels like it is intensifying. It is because new chi, new blood is pushing on it, new oxygen wants to come to it and you feel the pressure of that.

After completing this exercise, you may feel stiff, uncomfortable, etc., because you are becoming more aware of your pain body. Fear not, you are also clearing it out and cleaning it up!

Set your timer for five, ten, or fifteen minutes and give this one a try. I dare you!

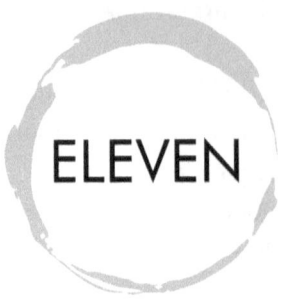

# ELEVEN

# THE WALL

"Have to keep go. No choice. Never ever give up." Tae Kwon Do Grandmaster - Kwon Jae Hwa

If you are a runner, you know what your wall is. If you are an avid distance hiker, a bicyclist, a triathlete, a Tae Kwon Do practitioner training with Grandmaster Kwon, etc., you know your wall. Whether you are an athlete or not, you have a wall that you will come up against now and then, depending on how much you are pushing the envelope of who you think you are.

Writers who are attempting to express themselves hit those walls and when they get stuck wrestling with one of them, they talk about it as writer's block. Mothers who work and/or take their kids all over town and/or go to the gym or practice yoga on the side know the wall.

It hits you at about 9 pm or whatever that magic hour is for you. These walls are internal, they are psychological, and they are sometimes described in the mainstream as blocks or barriers to success. Spiritual teachers describe them as blocks to your evolution. To success coaches, they are holding you back from living your best life.

High school and college students who push themselves in academics and sometimes in sports as well, regularly experience this wall. Some people are living right up against their wall all the time and some people cross it, go over it or through it, to find yet another wall. Motivational speakers attempt to motivate people to go over, under, or through those walls and preachers talk about the power of asking God or the Holy Spirit for help to dissolve those walls.

We can talk about these walls in conjunction with the power of belief, and we can talk about psychological self-doubt versus confidence, all of which is useful. Knowing, though, that your biggest obstacle is emotional, not mental, is extremely important. It is also very important for you to realize that the essence of who you are is never in question—you are its master, it becomes what you tell it to. Other people who question themselves will question you and challenge you and try and keep you down all day long if you let them, though.

Who am I? People are asking this all the time. The emotional answer is always that you are the collection of unfinished, unresolved emotional debris and its associated self-doubt and limited beliefs of your past telling you who you once were. This collection of information is based on unresolved previous experience, and has nothing to do with the essence of who you are. It cannot stop you from transmuting yourself and your life if you know what you are doing and practice doing it! Unless you agree with those emotions through identification, unawareness, and/or addiction and the associated mental postures that go with that, you have the power to free yourself from their bondage.

As a teacher of qigong, I think people could save themselves a lot of time and make quicker progress by realizing that at the heart of all their struggles lies a personal battle with lower-based emotions. These emotions include anger, greed, jealousy, self-doubt, confusion, guilt, and fear, to name a few. These emotions often present themselves as one collective mishmash of resistance. That resistance can be considered as part ego and part pain. Ego is often referred to as the false self. The false self is simply a record of information about who you think you are based on past experience.

When you identify with the false self and the past, pain is the result. Without even realizing it, most people think they are their past and, furthermore, they believe they are their emotions. The moment you think you are your emotions you are stuck, stagnating in your life, looping, and sometimes you will even feel paralyzed. These emotions are energetic in nature—it's all stored as energy and it all listens to your overall and consistent commands.

Whether you are a runner or not, this analogy will make sense to you metaphorically. A marathon runner hits walls throughout a race. If you are a marathoner, you likely know the walls. Maybe you hit your first wall at ten miles, the second at thirteen, the third at seventeen, and the last wall at about twenty-three miles.

Why does anyone hit a wall? Remember, it is emotional; it is a feeling thing. You are not going to hear a marathon runner (for the most part) say that they got to mile thirteen and simply had to quit because they got too emotional. Ninety-nine times out of a hundred, they will say they had to quit at whatever mile they had to quit at (which is a choice and subjective) because of the pain. They will say it was a pain in the ankle, a pain or cramp in the thigh, and that they just could not keep going.

Do you think that the winner of some marathon on some particular day had any pain? Did they still win? The name of the game is to push through pain without permanently injuring yourself. Only by pushing through pain, dissolving pain, transmuting emotion, stretching and evolving yourself can you grow and transcend your past.

You don't have to be a runner to learn to be familiar with pushing through pain. Anyone who's sat an extended meditation retreat or had a difficult labor or worked out hard physically or worked long hours to complete an important project is familiar with the experience.

Your life is like a series of mini-marathons. Those marathons, those life challenges, will either cause you to grow and evolve, building your stores of energy and power, or they will suck the life out of you.

If you are thinking about complaining right now about how difficult your life has been, don't! Wherever you are, pick yourself up and keep going, because this journey is about the evolution of the spirit! Your physical pain and your associated emotions and/or emotional pain cannot keep you. It reflects your hidden thoughts and it is all there to be worked through. Whether you know it or not you are one with all things. If you are one with all things, then your deepest thoughts influence all things. They influence your emotions, your physical health, your biology, your client's biology—you have influence over all of it. You can pretend otherwise, but you would be wrong.

Some people, myself included, believe in life before, after, and during death. If that's a belief you share, it makes it that much more important that you embrace this teaching. Keep moving through the challenges that come your way because they are there for you to evolve through. In Buddhist practices, for example, a Buddha does not become like the historical Buddha in one lifetime.

Professional marathon runners experience walls and pain, and that pain is emotional. They will never grow their discipline without going beyond these inner barriers. They have to learn to deal with, manage, overcome, and dissolve their pain. And unless they are injured, this is not done on the sidelines; it is done while running. They keep moving despite the physical pain, despite the emotional discomfort and challenge.

If you're a marathoner, you set your mind on the target of twenty-six miles and then you run. Then the pain comes. In general, when the pain becomes more intense it is because of the emotion that is rising.

Like a marathoner, you have to set intentions and focus on fulfilling them. That part is not so hard. When the pain comes, though, it gets hard. When you continue to try to move through any pain and it appears to be getting worse, it is because of the emotion that is coming with it. You can say "well, my hip was bone on bone," but I'm not talking about that type of injury. I'm talking about situations in which there is nothing medically wrong with you but you hurt. If you are a little sturdier, perhaps you push through even when you have a physical injury.

## A Personal Story: My Spartan Race in Black Mountain, North Carolina

When I did the Spartan race in Black Mountain, North Carolina, a couple of years ago we dropped into a river I ran across a deep section and split my shin open. It was a very deep wound and looked like it had been cut by a knife. It was very painful and I was shocked to see all the blood.

(I'm not being dramatic or graphic, just trying to make the point that even in extreme physical and emotional discomfort it is possible to transcend the walls. If I can do it in extreme conditions, you sure as heck should be able to do it in less extreme situations!) So I looked down, saw the blood, felt the pain and kept going. I said to myself, "Nothing happened here." I said to existence "Fix it!" I had no intention of quitting this race.

Mid-race the quad in the leg I injured began locking up and seizing— it was like a bag of bricks. Once again, it came calling to me. Once again, I applied these principles. I told myself this was a mental idea about an emotional experience and that it was not as physical as I was imagining. After several minutes of continuing to put one foot in front of the other my leg stopped seizing. I continued on and finished the race.

I finished very well overall and conquered all the obstacles I encountered. When my wife and daughter saw me, they said, "Oh my God what did you do to your leg?" We all headed to the emergency medical booth.

So when I got to the EMTs, they cleaned my wound, and said I needed stiches. I chose to go home and have my wife and daughter bandage it, and they gave it a lot of love and attention. I once again said to existence "Fix it!" Today I hardly have a trace of a scar there—it cleaned up and healed very nicely for me. I never thought once again about any kind of bacterial infection. I did not talk to biology in that way and I never had a problem with it again.

Now I am not suggesting that you go to these extremes, but, again, if I can do it with extremes maybe you can do it with something less intense. The pain in your life in your literal or metaphorical race is your disbelief saying, "I cannot do this thing that I said I was going to do." If you quit doing something that you really wanted to do, you quit not just because you do not believe you can do it. You quit because of the pain! It's too damn uncomfortable to step up and exercise your new and improved belief over the body, because in order to do it, there is a birthing process. That's why people quit. It's not just that they did not believe they could do it—they could not do it because it freaking hurt too much! This is an emotional wall, an emotional hurdle, and you must overcome it in order to truly move forward in your life.

The beauty of qigong is that you are very, very unlikely to hurt yourself doing it and yet it provides you a similar challenge to running a race when it comes to healing your body and conquering your emotional past. It actually offers the best of many worlds.

What if I told you that there are ways to get through your mini metaphorical marathons that would help you accomplish your goals and reduce the amount of pain you experience? Many of the exercises I've introduced you to accomplish exactly that! There are ways to work with your beliefs, your energy, your body, and your energy system that will propel you forward without ever having to run at all. There are qigong techniques that offer the benefits of running without the running. Of course, for those of you who like to run or go to the gym, but can't because of some pain or injury, I have a new word and practice for you—it's called qigong!

## Depression

Let's use depression as an example. Do you think running would help your depression? Yes, it would, but maybe you are not able to run or running just isn't your thing.

Or you are depressed because you like to run but your ankles and/or knees or hips are bothering you. Or maybe you have a story that says, "My knees hurt because of all my years of running—at least according to my doctor." If that is you, listen up.

One of the best and most healing aspects of running is breath exchange—the release of carbon dioxide and the intake of oxygen. Remember that depression is a mood. It is biology, and you can change that biology. You can try not to feed it, you can try fighting it, but that doesn't work. You can give up and surrender to it, but that doesn't work either.

Try something different—change your thinking. "I can't right now," you say. Ok, fine; change your breathing! "I can't do that." Yes you can!

If you change your breathing through breath of fire, through qigong movement practices, you will change your level of depression, period. If you are depressed, that is your marathon. Keeping up with your life, that is your marathon. You are not a victim of your biology and its chemicals, natural or otherwise. It may seem like you are and it may seem hopeless, but hopeless is an attitude.

What if depression is just a cloud cover? What if depression is not the essence of who you are, but rather an expression of energetic and emotional pain? Your depression may feel like it will be with you forever, but it can last only as long as you persist in thinking that you are your depression.

What if you could begin to observe your depression as an energetic and emotional wall and breathe through it? You could with practice. What if you could think through it? You could with practice.

## Anxiety

Anxiety is the flip side of depression. Some teachers like to say that depression is a belief in the past and anxiety is a fear of the future. Well, that is really the same thing, isn't it?

Here's the deal, though. You are not your past, and the future is yet to be determined based on how you handle the now. Meanwhile, there is this wall.

Here is a very, very important point—this wall cannot be reasoned with! If you want it to change, you cannot mumble to it. If you want to change it, which you have the power to do, you cannot just sit there and let it talk to you! You have to realize who you are.

So who are you really? I love how Tony Robbins talks about becoming "the voice." I love how he talks about the difference between a mantra and an incantation. A mantra can be mumbled. An incantation is loud! You step into the mindset that you are the voice now! And then you tell that little annoying voice what is what.

I tripped over this when I was younger. I just could not stand it anymore—I was depressed, I was anxious, and all the while I was listening to this bully in my head. One day I took him outside and I yelled back at him. I mean I let him have it! He seemed to get quiet. Then he came back louder. The second time I cut his head off; as a modern peaceful warrior, I cut his head off in the name of peace. I learned something very profound that day, and I have never stopped letting that voice in my head know who the boss is: "I am the supreme grandmaster creator of my personal reality and I have total dominion over my biology, my ego, and my life!" Many years after that experience, I found that Tony Robbins, in his own way, discovered that same thing many years before I did and look what he has done with it!

Qigong and meditation masters agree with quantum physicists: "You are the observer." What does that mean?

It means you have the power to take a step back. It means the wall, the cloud, the mood, is not who you are. It is energy—stuck emotion—and you can walk, run, fly, breathe, or swim through it. You can go into a meditative state in which you are the observer and become so still in your watchfulness and alertness that you begin to realize you are not a mood. You are not an emotion; you are the awareness of that emotion. You realize that you cannot be stopped by walls that you dis-identify with and begin to observe from above. The wall, the depression, the anxiety are not at all indicative of who you are, not if you identify with the "observer" of that emotional content.

## Qigong Practice: Breathing

Be still physically. Either sit, stand, or lie down. Be very still. See if you can sense your breath and your underlying emotions. Be very still and begin to observe them. Now whisper to yourself, "Be." Then pause. Then again "Be." Pause, then whisper, "Be still." This is an intention that you are expressing or suggesting to yourself. Now say "Be still and know." Know what? This means tap into knowing, tap into your own intuition, tap into divine intelligence. Then pause a few moments. Then say, "Be. Be still. Be still and know." Then pause. Then say "Be, be still and know I am." Then pause. Then whisper to yourself "Be. Be still. Know. Know that I am. I am the I am. I am the light."

This is an old mantra that can be used to calm your mind and body and tap you into a deeper level of your own inner being and the knowingness that lives inside you. This is a means to discover what the Buddhists call your true nature.

If, however, you do tell yourself you are the mood, your experience of it and its associated mindset becomes more solid and "real." Why? Because by your very nature you are an amplifier; what you focus on gets bigger energetically. As your energy becomes more and more light and buoyant, you generate greater happiness. As you focus on anger, your energy becomes more and more angry. You have the power to amplify good feelings and bad ones, so choose wisely.

You are not your emotions, you are not your pain body, you are not your mood, you are not your walls—those are emotional. When you feel down, you can try talking yourself out of it, but that is challenging to do unless you have a lot of practice. You can, though, use a power walk and a power talk to get you headed in the right direction.

If you are a runner, you can go for a long run until you break through that wall. Sometimes you can run for thirteen miles and still come home feeling depleted and doubting yourself.

Whatever your current challenge is, qigong practice, especially techniques like enhanced tree meditation practiced in stillness and/or in conjunction with the breath of fire, will begin to show you that you are not the emotion! What do you think happens to your self-doubt then?

## Qigong Exercise: Breath of Fire

Stand in a natural stance and relax your arms and shoulders. Breathe in and out through your nose. In and out, in and out; repeat. You should see and feel your belly rising. Don't allow your chest to move up and down. Focus on the belly. It takes practice, but give it a try.

What happens to your limited thinking, your bad mood, or the bully in your head? Simple—it goes away for a while. It goes away until your subconscious mind starts thinking limited thoughts, creating a limited mood, which eventually reveals the emotional wall again. If you identify with that wall and that mood, it gets worse again. If you keep it up you begin to attract people and events that further reveal the emotional struggle. They show up as problems.

So, to break the cycle, do the practice! Knowing how to do it is not enough; you must do it! Over time, you will see different external results that help you gain confidence and pride in yourself and your accomplishments.

Even after you know and experience this, you can and will easily forget it. As great and revelatory as this information is—and it is—it is mostly worthless without an associated practice like qigong. You have to have the knowledge, but you also have to have discipline to practice.

Many people have a qigong practice on some level, but do not have the deeper wisdom that goes with the practice, so it can only go so far and do so much. Some people have a grasp of the intellectual and spiritual ideas but no practice to help them actualize them. Most people, of course, have neither of these key ingredients to personal transformation and so they rely on hope. Hope will not heal your body or pay the bills, though.

Where hope leaves off, practice picks up, and where practice leads is to the revelation that you are not the wall, you are not its associated mood, you are not its self-doubt or confusion. You can exercise and be the will, the part of your mind that is bigger than any wall, any emotion, any limited belief and you can use that power to change how you feel. When you change how you feel, you will believe it—you will believe in your health, you will believe in your vitality and well-being, and when you do that, your body and the rest of your life will follow.

## Masters

Using your will to overcome walls is an approach that you may or may not resonate with. Spiritual masters also suggest another way. Their way involves no yelling and no running up mountains (although some masters do that too). It involves the practice of no mind/no reaction, yet total observation of the emotional wall, the mood, the pain body. As you become the observer of that emotion, and as you begin to watch it without reacting to it, without freaking out about it or stuffing it, then you begin to realize "Hey I am watching this. If I am watching it, I am not it. I am the observer of it!"

These masters also refer to this watcher or observer as the "I am." The I am is not the emotion, it is the watcher of the emotion. It is still, despite the chaos. Runners can find this place of mind, and—in my opinion— it's likely what allows them to set an intention such as running a certain distance in a certain period of time at a certain pace and not stopping for a moment despite emotional and physical pain. Those who stay in the realm of the observer are practicing being in a state of no mind. The best runners do this all the time. They may or may not call it a spiritual place, but it is.

Whether you're a runner or not, you can train the part of you that has the power to observe and watch so that you are not distracted by physical and/or emotional pain. If you have a particular goal that you would like to achieve—finishing a marathon (literally or metaphorically), for example—then, just like a physical runner, you have to focus on the finish line at different points along the way. Just as important, though, is that you must be present with every step and you must deal with the emotional blocks, which are ghosts from the past trying to stop you, telling you that you cannot do it for a million different reasons. This past can be transcended and qigong can help you to do it physically, mentally, and even in the presence of the inner beast of your emotional past.

Your life challenges will appear or disappear, depending on how you handle that wall. Are you expanding yourself energetically and emotionally in the face of your internal wall and its associated challenges, or are you contracting yourself and shrinking from opportunities that arise?

When you think the wall is you, you will feel hopeless, lost, tired, and abandoned—you will want to quit. If you think others are keeping you down, you will blame them. All of this activity causes you to contract rather than expand, so the wall is further solidified. If you know the wall is emotional and you know you are not the emotion, you can identify more closely with the higher mind, the will, and power through it, perhaps in a seated, quiet, defenseless practice of meditation. Or you can power walk and power talk until you change your biology so that your energy field expands exponentially. Both are effective paths to the same destination.

Remember that you can't just dabble, however. You have to choose your transformation tools and work at it!

## *Qigong Practice: Using Laughter as the Best Medicine*

The wall is serious. Many professional athletes think so. People who are ill and working to heal themselves think so too.

I am a firm believer in physical and metaphysical cross training. It can keep you from getting bored and gives you a better chance to stay active and make progress toward your self-improvement goals without burning out.

I am going to give you one more exercise that can help you remain the observer of a challenge rather than getting caught up in it. It can help you dissolve the wall in a moment and rise above it. This exercise is also good for your body, even if you are just faking it.

Many studies have shown that the mind can't tell the difference between the real and the imaginary. You can use this quirk to your advantage—any situation can be lightened, depending on how you look at it and what you do with it.

So don't forget to smile once in a while and don't forget to laugh. You do not have to wait for a good movie to laugh and you do not have to wait until your qigong practice or your run is over to smile. Smile while practicing qigong. Smile slightly while running and watch how much easier it makes the hills. Laugh for the health of it. Laugh when you feel you cannot go on. Watch your ego react to your audacity to laugh in the face of emotional turmoil.

Did you know that when you laugh you literally turn on internal medicine in your body and brain? You do, by stimulating the production of serotonin, "the happy hormone." Start laughing and your body is going to make more of it. Smile and you use all kinds of muscles in your face and your whole body begins to secrete powerful healing elixirs. The part of your mind that says, "I cannot laugh for no reason," is the same part of your mind that is making you sick. Maybe it is time to stop taking that part of the mind so seriously:

- Set the timer for one minute and belly laugh!
- If you need more of a boost check out the laughter meditations on my YouTube channel.

I discussed smiling and laughter practice in CHAPTER SIX: MASTER YOUR MOOD, but it's worth mentioning again. Learning to laugh for no reason is a skill. It is even more of a skill when you can laugh when you're go through a rough patch. When you laugh in such a way that says "Ha ha ha as if this could ever really be a problem. Life is unlimited and in my unlimited-ness I laugh because this little tiny miniscule problem is already resolved!" That takes confidence, but it's a confidence you can build.

There are different ways to go under, around, over, or through your walls. Learn the skills and practice the skills—these are life skills with the potential to help you immensely! Try them on for size—you have nothing to lose and everything to gain. You may fail many times, but the time will come when you succeed, and you will be on your way to a higher state of living and being!

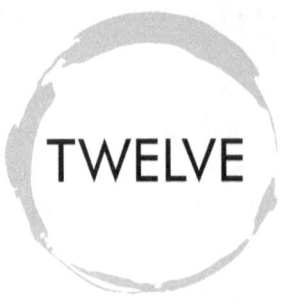

# TWELVE

# THE POWER OF PRACTICING STILLNESS

---

"In mindfulness one is not only restful and happy, but alert and awake. Meditation is not evasion; it is a serene encounter with reality." Thich Nhat Hanh

---

You now have many teachings and practices that will change your life if you do them. They will teach you about the power that lives in you and that is the real you. Remember that energy cannot be destroyed; it can only be changed from one form to another. Throw a stone in a pond and what do you get? Ripples. Those ripples exemplify the law of karma or what I like to call the boomerang effect. You are throwing boomerangs in your life left and right. When you throw them without mindfulness, they will then come back and hit you in the head later. Nobody else did that to you, you did it. Own it and throw some new boomerangs with new intention.

Change your energy and you will change your life. Knowledge is key and yet the greatest knowledge lives within us. Jesus, Buddha, and other sages have told us this, but many of us keep looking outside ourselves for the key to our happiness. Consequently, like the proverbial carrot dangled just out of reach of the horse's face, true happiness seems to elude most of us. Jesus said that the Kingdom of Heaven lives within us. The Buddha left us meditation. In various areas of the Orient, it is common for masters and sages and gurus to teach stillness practice.

In the West, many do not have time for stillness. Really?

What if you knew without a doubt that your energy field is attracting very specific people, places, events, etc. to you and that unless you change that energy field from the inside out, your life will remain as it is; same stuff, different day."

What if you knew without a doubt that if you changed your mind-body field through stillness practice you could attract better people, places, situations, and circumstances? Would you take the time to do that?

What if you understood that there are no outer shortcuts, only inner ones, and that the work has to be done inside you before you will see the change outside? Would you make the time to make the necessary changes?

So many people say that they cannot afford the time. We would be wise to make some time for these practices, because the practices can create more time for us. Fewer problems, struggles, and loose ends lead to more quality time.

What if I gave you a practice that that would provide answers and solutions to your current struggles, propel you forward, and take less than five minutes a day? Would you want to know what it is?

What if I told you that you do not even have to break a sweat? What if I also told you that it will only take a little effort to break through this wall of yours? What if I told you the goal of the exercise was to set down your resistance altogether?

Interested?

This exercise is not going to get you in great physical shape or tone your muscles. It will, however, not only answer your questions and give you solutions to problems, but also reduce your stress and cause vital life hormones and healing agents to be secreted in your body. It is a great practice for reducing stress, overcoming your internal and external walls, and feeding the body blood, chi, and lymph. This can be done in lieu of exercise, on your days off from working out or when you are injured.

There are times to move and times to be loud, times to be quiet and times to be reserved. This exercise is potent. I saved it for last because it is one of the simplest exercises in principle, but one of the most difficult to follow through on. I believe, though, that if more people experienced and understood the power of stillness, how it works, and the many benefits it provides, more people would do it more often.

## Qigong Exercise: Standing Tree Meditation

There are many different styles of stillness practice. One is standing qigong meditation, also known as standing tree meditation. When you practice standing tree meditation, you simply stand with the feet roughly shoulder width apart and your hands hanging at your sides. Your fingers stay open and relaxed. Close your eyes, unless you're more comfortable with them open. If you leave them open, pick a point in front of you and fix on it with a steady, relaxed gaze.

When you take this standing position, you are setting an intention for stillness. Stillness practice gathers exponential subtle energy to you that is otherwise dissipated by looking around, moving your body, and allowing the world to distract you. Practicing standing tree meditation is also a practice of inward seeking, looking within. This kind of practice can conjure up all kinds of ideas about what you might find when you go looking through the closet.

In psychotherapy, for example, you would go looking in the closet to uncover past, possibly traumatic events. Even in life coaching sessions, you would look through the closet to some degree. This is a very different approach than what I'm talking about here, although it is one that I recommend having in your personal transformation arsenal.

Through stillness practice, you bring various walls into awareness. Just like the runner who practices facing his or her walls all the way up the mountain, in this practice you stay with your wall and watch it dissolve. Unlike the runner, though, this practice is all about stillness. In this practice, you can discover a deeper level of who you are, what you are, and what life is.

The ego, the monkey mind, the record of your past, your biological record, your brain, your neural net, your beliefs, your identifications, and your emotions do not like to be observed. This is why most of us are regularly trying to distract ourselves from ourselves.

The monkey mind hates being physically still and will not like your attempts to quiet its nonsense, its bullying, its incessant noise, its beliefs, its mental postures, etc. It typically does not like it when you stand like a tree for no apparent reason for five or ten or sixty minutes at a time, let alone every morning for thirty days in a row. It sees absolutely no value in stillness practice, which should tell you something!

The monkey mind is okay with exhaustion and sleep and discomfort and distraction and confusion and pain, but not stillness. Stillness brings awareness. Awareness has the power to dissolve exhaustion, discomfort, pain, anger, etc. Physically, this practice will open meridians, chakras, blood flow, and lymph flow very profoundly. This is the power behind stillness practice.

Standing tree meditation takes some getting used to and even your monkey mind will accept it after you practice it ten or twenty times. If you manage to do that, there are many deeper levels of the practice I could introduce you to.

These types of poses are used by the military, and typically include some type of arm activity—holding the position of a cross for four hours, for example. This standing tree meditation practice that I am sharing with you differs in that there is less of an external effort and the energy is used to enhance the subtle internal experience. This has a very potent healing effect on the physical body.

From a traditional Chinese medicine standpoint, this practice opens up the kidneys and contributes to jing (essence) development, a potent life force that gives rise to chi energy. In general, though, standing like a tree produces extra and even excess energy. This energy builds in the lower belly and expands into your energy system, expanding the energy as well as consciousness itself.

When your consciousness is identified in the lower belly with the physical, mental, and emotional realms, your awareness is limited to those domains and remains unaware of the metaphysical aspects of who you are. Unless the chi builds, unless the mind sits and gathers energy, lets the energy rise, and transmutes the energy from metaphorical lead to metaphorical gold, from heaviness to lighter energy, the mind remains limited in its awareness of itself. Your problems cannot be surmounted through the same energy that created them—you have to find a way to gather more energy to yourself to tackle the challenges at hand.

Take the Navy SEAL who is holding a boat above his head after getting no sleep, eating no food, running thirty miles, and swimming ten. He may have the energy to hold the boat for five minutes; let's say that is the longest he has ever done it. If he has to do it for ten minutes—twice as long as he has ever had to do it—where will that energy come from? The energy must be generated and created or he might collapse. So the pose, the posture, the breathing, and mindset he holds during his training generates fuel to enable his body do what his body needs to do, as long as he does not give up.

This is one example of how and why the body-brain-energy field can and does generate energy. When you do the stillness practice of standing tree meditation without your arms held high, great energy is generated and, because there is no boat to hold over your head, there is less distraction. In that lack of distraction, you can achieve the awareness that you are the awareness, not the body and not the emotion; you are energy and awareness combined. If you prefer the term watcher or observer or that which is termed no mind, they work as descriptions, too. In order to surmount these walls, these emotions, these internal and external noes, there has to be a master who says, "I am in charge here and no wind will move me, I am immovable." You have to practice that attitude one time, two times, ten times, and the more you practice it, the more you can become that master.

In that place of centered-ness, stillness, the wind will blow, your emotions will rise, your pain will come to the surface. It will sometimes feel like something has you by the Achilles heel; you will feel that internal "no." Understand that when you take a stance against your ego, with its naysaying and bullying, you are not only challenging it in that moment, but you are facing all the issues going on in your life at once. Physicists say that your quantum field goes with you wherever you go. Your whole life goes with you wherever you go. It may be invisible but you are connected to it and you feel it.

When you take a still pose, you begin to speak to it without words. You begin to speak to it with presence. Many masters say you are that presence. Presence observes. It is still in the face of any storm and it has the power to dissolve all storms and bring a deep internal calm. That internal calm can provide solutions. It has answers that do not argue with the noise that your bullying ego makes in your head. Many masters say that truth needs no defense; it does not compete. It is still.

Would you move for an ant that was trying to bully you if you knew you were a giant? Hell, no, you wouldn't! So what is the issue? The issue is that you think this noise is bigger than you are, more important than you are, more together than you are—but it isn't. So what does this suggest that you are up against? Its belief isn't it? Belief that you are the little mind- the false self rather then the presence that is still magnitude watching quietly in the background. You can identify with one or the other but not both simultaneously.

In CHAPTER SEVEN: PRIMARY THINKING VERSUS SECONDARY THINKING, I said that secondary thinking was your biology talking, your ego flapping when you wake up in the morning and your body telling you that you are tired. I said that you could use primary thinking and say, "I am the supreme grandmaster creator of my personal reality and I say I have tons of energy, tons of it!" In such a command, you are reprogramming your body; in that moment, you are running the show.

With stillness practice, you are using an even higher level of primary thinking—presence itself. You are using that silence in the background and that background houses the wisdom of all the ages.

You can become the supreme grandmaster creator of your personal reality by adopting an attitude of being bigger than your tiredness or the voices in your head. With practice, you can become the commanding officer, telling your biology what to do.

In stillness practice, the message is very different. It's as if you're allowing the Source in you, the Holy Spirit in you, the voice for the universal life force or the presence in you to have a face-to-face silent transmission that affects this nonsense monkey mind, this noise, this lethargy and sleep, or this anxiety you feel. In such a practice, your job is to stay out of the way. Let higher mind have a conversation in stillness with the bully. You are simply the observer.

Here is another way of thinking about it, which involves inspiration, solutions, prayers answered, problems solved, and universal and divine intelligence downloaded. Can this be done in just five minutes a day? Yes, in fact that is where it must begin because it requires some discipline.

## Qigong Practice: Standing Tree Meditation

Here is a twenty-one-day stillness meditation challenge you can do in only five minutes a day:

- Get a calendar and a timer.
- Look at twenty-one days going forward.
- Mark the start date and end date.
- Set the timer.
- Stand with feet shoulder width apart.
- Do not move.
- Bend knees slightly.
- Keep your feet where you placed them.
- Keep your eyes closed unless you get dizzy or otherwise uncomfortable.
- If eyes are open, look with a relaxed gaze in front of you (do not look around).
- Do not scratch your face even if it itches. Every time you do, your monkey mind gains power because it got you to move and dissipate the energy momentum.
- For a more challenging practice elevate the arms as pictured below!
- Do this for twenty-one days, five minutes per day.
- If you miss one day, make it up by doing ten minutes the next day; it's better to stick to five minutes each day, though.

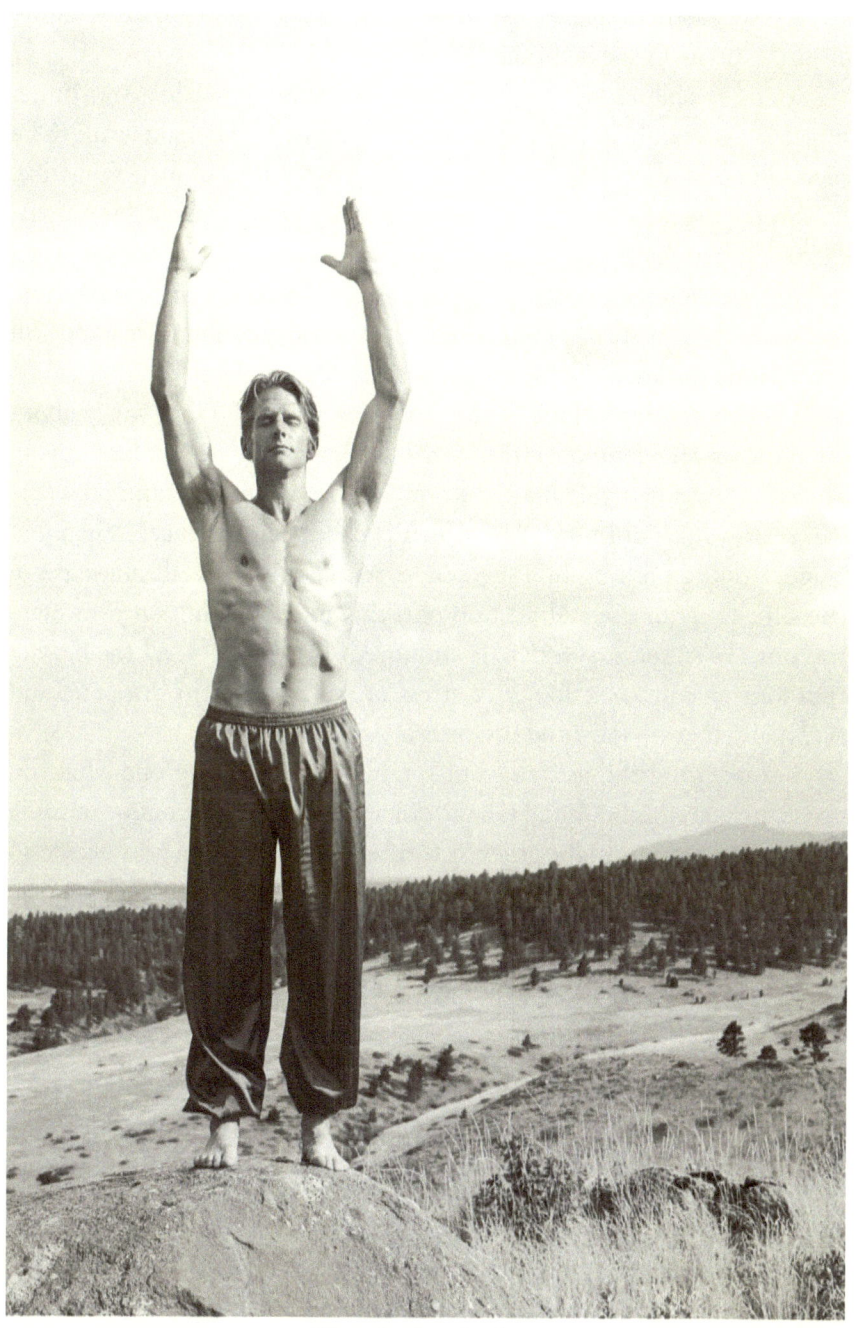

*Photo By: Lisa Siciliano*

If everyone realized what this accomplishes and all of the problems it solves, everybody would do it! You can do it outside on top of a tree stump or just at home in the bedroom.

Many people are looking for outer shortcuts only; this is an inner shortcut that can help you create outer shortcuts. If you really want to be successful and want to see for yourself the great benefit of such a practice, do this for twenty-one days, and every couple of days make a few journal entries. What challenges do you have? Before each practice session, ask a specific question about a challenge you would like to resolve or something you would like to create. Then do not answer the question. Just stand still and assume the answer will come in a silent transmission!

Do not wait for or look for big booming voices. Do not worry about the noise of your monkey mind; relax and let it face the absolute in you! There is a secret here that masters know. Within stillness, within presence, within you lives all knowledge, which is called omniscience. When you practice doing nothing in a meditative sense, you allow all nonsense to rise, all chatter to rise and, instead of trying to deal with it on your own, you observe stillness, you remain unmoved. In that place, all the heavier emotions or pain or lethargy or stress or worry begin to dissipate, and eventually they dissolve and disappear.

I expect great things from you! You may want to go beyond what you can learn from this book and take advantage of our live and online training opportunities. You might go even further in the training and decide to become one of our Certified Qigong instructors and/or Certified Medical Qigong Practitioners. You can change the world, starting with your own!

# AFTERWORD

Qigong is a practice. It is traditionally defined as the skilled cultivation of universal life force or chi. Chi can be thought of as energy. Everything you do either adds to your life force energy reserves or depletes them. When you have a lot of energy, you are powerful. When you have little energy, your power is weakened.

Remember, power in this context means your ability to influence yourself, your body, and your surroundings, including people, situations, circumstances and events. I am not simply a teacher of the exercise of qigong, which, in and of itself, may be a fantastic practice. I am someone who lives in the West, is busy, runs a business, is writing a book, is filming qigong videos, and is creating online medical qigong courses for health professionals, including acupuncturists and massage therapists. I have sought out and received approval from the National Certification Commission for Acupuncture and Oriental Medicine, the National Certification Board for Therapeutic Massage and Bodywork, and the Florida, Texas, and California Acupuncture Boards.

I have a psychology degree, I was an emergency medical technician, and I have three black belts and a great deal of advanced martial arts training. I travel the country teaching seminars to lay people and professionals. I have a daughter who I home school. I have a private healing and coaching practice, and I offer long distance healing clinics. My wife, Tanya Mei-Tai Coon, an acupuncturist with a deep grounding in Oriental medicine, and I have created a certification program for qigong instructors and medical qigong practitioners.

I am not just marketing to you here, I am asking you a question—what do you think it takes for someone to do all that? Answer, it takes energy! No energy, no power, no power, and you have no ability to influence your life! Whether you are more concerned about your body, your job, your business, or your income potential, do not forget this—you will need energy and a lot of it!

If you are a practitioner and/or caretaker in a profession like acupuncture, massage, nursing, etc., then you need energy to keep going with what you have begun. If you are giving to others all day in your job and then going home to a family, wow! I know how much energy that takes.

So many people cannot even take care of themselves and then some are brave enough to also take on the care of others. Regardless of your personal situation, if you need energy and if you want to influence your outer world and get ahead of the game rather than always being behind that eight ball, I have given you multiple tools, multiple practices to begin that effort.

I am offering you these writings as a means to educate and inspire you. Remember that everything you do, or say, or think, or feel, or ask, or demand, or contemplate, or challenge, or fear either gives you energy or it robs you of energy. If you were to create a list for yourself on your mirror for the week and have a column that said energy in and another column that said energy out, you would be able to see what your energy balance looks like. Remember also that there are things that require more energy input like qigong practice, like running, like going for a power walk and exercising your voice and your power thinking over your biology. That takes energy. It does. What you put in, though, you will get back exponentially from such practices.

Remember there will be internal walls, emotional walls, physical walls, and mental walls that you will experience inside yourself and that you will watch as they take form outside yourself. If you want power and dominion over these internal and external challenges, you need a practice. If you are an ultramarathon runner, you do not necessarily need qigong, although it would help you immensely with your recovery. You might also benefit from the idea of power walking and power talking over your body. If, though, you are someone who does not even like exercise, or you like it but do not have time, or exercise is nice, but it does not really help you transcend the internal obstacles you are facing, then this book, this teaching is for you. If you seek the metaphysical, this book is also for you.

If you choose to integrate qigong exercise and practice into your life and use it to gather energy to you, you will increase your energy levels and improve your health. If you further build upon that energy by power walking, talking, and thinking and begin replacing the old negative habits with new ones, you will begin to gather even greater energy and begin to become powerful in your ability to influence your inner and outer world.

If you decide to learn qigong from us and become a certified qigong instructor, you can get paid while you practice. You can make money doing something you love and you can gain greater momentum from that energy and power. If you decide to learn the medical qigong practices we teach and/or become certified as a medical qigong practitioner, you can make significantly more money with significantly less burnout than you can, for example, with a traditional massage practice.

Practice is only hard if you do not enjoy it. More than eight million people enjoy qigong practice every day. Walking and talking over your biology is all about building your confidence. No one expects you to begin with that confidence, but you will develop it as your practice strengthens.

Martial arts are also a great practice for developing confidence, but many martial arts require fighting, sparring, and self-defense, which are much more likely to cause injury. Qigong is safe, yet it embodies many of the same great qualities of martial arts without the need for excessive combat, conflict, or injury. I love martial arts, but they are not for everyone. Qigong, on the other hand, is something anybody can do, at any age, in any condition.

Unlike everyday exercise, qigong taps into the extraordinary. I see it often, with many people. Read some, watch the videos, come to a live workshop and practice with us. We would love you to be part of our qigong family. I am available to my students in many different ways, so watch me, practice along with me, come to a workshop, or hire me as a personal life coach.

At the time of this writing, I am offering weekly classes in Wilmington, North Carolina and travelling around the country to teach in various North Carolina & Florida locations as well as Boulder- Denver Colorado.

Through these qigong practices and a larger-than-life attitude, I will help you go over, under, around, or through that next set of obstacles. I will help you define a destiny that serves you and others simultaneously.

Together we can make the world better!

Best of luck and power to you!
Practice! Practice! Practice!
David J. Coon

www.ingramcontent.com/pod-product-compliance
Lightning Source LLC
Chambersburg PA
CBHW030445290526
45786CB00001B/449